# DEFIANT TEENS

# DEFIANT TEENS

## A Clinician's Manual
## for Assessment and Family Intervention

**RUSSELL A. BARKLEY**
**GWENYTH H. EDWARDS**
**ARTHUR L. ROBIN**

THE GUILFORD PRESS
New York   London

Printed in the United States of America

This book is printed on acid-free paper.

Last digit is print number:   9   8   7   6   5   4

**Library of Congress Cataloging-in-Publication Data**

Barkley, Russell A., 1949–
    Defiant teens: a clinician's manual for assessment and family
training / Russell A. Barkley, Gwenyth H. Edwards, and Arthur L.
Robin.
        p.   cm.
    Includes bibliographical references and index.
    ISBN 1-57230-440-5 (pbk.)
    1. Oppositional defiant disorder in adolescence.   2. Family
psychotherapy.   I. Edwards, Gwenyth H.   II. Robin, Arthur L.
III. Title.
RJ506.066B37   1999
616.89'00835—dc21                                         98-52420
                                                              CIP

# About the Authors

**Russell A. Barkley, PhD**, is director of psychology and professor of psychiatry and neurology at the University of Massachusetts Medical School, Worcester. He is a diplomate in both clinical psychology and clinical neuropsychology (ABPP and ABCN) and is the author of more than 150 scientific papers and book chapters dealing primarily with ADHD. He has also authored or coedited 13 books and created 6 professional videotapes on ADHD and defiant children. He has served as president of the Section of Clinical Child Psychology of the American Psychological Association and president of the International Society for Research in Child and Adolescent Psychopathology.

**Gwenyth H. Edwards, PhD**, is chief of the ADHD Child and Adolescent Clinic at the University of Massachusetts Medical Center, Worcester. Dr. Edwards is an assistant professor of psychiatry and pediatrics and a licensed psychologist. She has provided the clinical leadership on two treatment outcome studies for children and adolescents diagnosed with both Attention-Deficit/Hyperactivity Disorder and disruptive behavior disorders. As a colleague of Dr. Barkley's, Dr. Edwards has provided diagnostic evaluations for over 2,000 children and teens with behavioral, academic, and emotional problems. She has also provided training for educators, mental health professionals, psychology graduate students, psychiatry and pediatric residents, and a variety of visiting professionals from around the United States and the world.

**Arthur L. Robin, PhD**, is professor of psychiatry and behavioral neurosciences and pediatrics at Wayne State University School of Medicine and chief of psychology at Children's Hospital of Michigan in Detroit. Director of the Developmental Neurosciences Research Division of the Department of Psychiatry and Behavioral Neurosciences, Dr. Robin has extensive clinical and research experience conducting evaluations and treatment with ADHD, eating disorders, and family conflict in children, adolescents, and adults. In addition to many research articles, chapters, grants, and videos, he has written two books, *Negotiating Parent–Adolescent Conflict: A Behavioral–Family Systems Approach* (Guilford Press, 1989) and *ADHD in Adolescents: Diagnosis and Treatment* (Guilford Press, 1998).

# Preface

This clinician's manual for assessment and family intervention builds upon two earlier programs of research and clinical work. First, it represents an extension of Russell Barkley's previous, long-term, programmatic work developing an effective program for training parents of defiant children (Barkley, 1987, 1997b). And second, it represents our efforts to enhance the efficacy of that program when extended to working with families of adolescents having Oppositional Defiant Disorder (ODD) by modifying those earlier procedures and, more importantly, combining them with a family therapy program developed by Arthur Robin and Sharon Foster (Robin & Foster, 1989). That family therapy program is known as problem-solving communication training (PSCT), and has been shown previously to be of assistance in clinical work with families experiencing significant parent–adolescent conflicts.

The combination of these programs into a single family training manual is a natural one, given that each targets somewhat different aspects of family functioning in their common goal to improve parent–teen relationships and teen adjustment. Barkley's program for defiant children concentrates on giving parents sufficient skills to manage disruptive, defiant, and noncompliant child behavior through controlling the antecedents and consequences of those forms of child misconduct. This exclusive focus on parents' competence at child management is sensible for families with young children, because parents have greater control and influence over young children's behavior and well-being. In addition, young children are not yet psychologically, socially, or legally autonomous of their parents' guidance and influence. As children enter adolescence, however, they are increasingly less influenced by their parents' guidance and their family environment in general. Adolescents are rapidly developing a psychological sense of autonomy and individuation from their parents and families. Thus interventions, to be effective, must focus on the adolescent's, as well as his or her parents', need for interactional management, and so must make the adolescent an active participant in any family change program. The PSCT program originally developed by Robin and Foster does just that: it concentrates on training both the parents and the adolescent in more effective ways of negotiating conflicts, resolving problems or disputes, developing more effective communication styles, and changing unreasonable beliefs about other family members that may adversely influence specific interactions.

Like Barkley's earlier clinical manual, this book sets forth a sequence of procedures for training parents in adolescent behavior-management skills that Barkley has employed over the past 20 years of clinical research and practice with a variety of behavior-disordered children and adolescents. These procedures have been modified somewhat for the developmental characteristics of adolescence, and constitute the first half of this family training manual (Steps 1–9). Only the parents attend these training sessions, the focus of which is to provide parents with more effective tools for interacting with their teenager and specifically for managing the adolescent's noncompliant or defiant behavior. The family training program of Robin and Foster then comprises the second half of this family treatment program (Steps 10–18), the sessions of which are attended by both the parents and the adolescent. Focus shifts toward helping each of the family members develop more effective problem-solving, negotiation, and communication skills with each other, while helping each to reframe and correct any unreasonable beliefs that may be unearthed in the therapeutic process.

The chapters in Part I are adapted from Barkley's (1997) manual for child behavior-management training. Additional information on the nature of oppositional and conduct problems in adolescents has also been inserted into this part of the manual. Included in the manual are not only the step-by-step instructions for conducting each session of this family training program, but also specific methods for the clinical assessment of adolescents exhibiting defiant behavior or ODD, a condition that is associated in the majority of cases with Attention-Deficit/Hyperactivity Disorder (ADHD) and sometimes Conduct Disorder (CD). Tools for evaluating the nature, diversity, and severity of parent–adolescent conflicts are also provided, as are some tools for evaluating parental psychological adjustment, especially parental ODD and ADHD, in view of the hereditary nature of the latter and familial commonality of the former.

The program described here owes much to an ongoing series of research projects conducted by Barkley over the past decade and funded by the National Institute of Mental Health (NIMH). Those projects have attempted to evaluate the efficacy of each of these two training programs separately and, more recently, the value of their combination into a single treatment program for teens having both ADHD and ODD, many of whom also had CD. Those research programs were funded by NIMH Grant No. MH41583 to Barkley, who expresses his gratitude here for that support. Gwen Edwards served as project manager and clinical therapist over the past 3 years for this program of research, and Arthur Robin has served as a consultant to this project throughout. The opinions expressed here, however, are entirely those of the authors and do not necessarily represent those of the Institute.

Parts of this program also owe much to the stimulating, heuristic, and collaborative discussions we have had over the years with others trained in the original programs, including Sharon Foster, Charles Cunningham, Eric Mash, and Eric Ward. They have been most instrumental in modifying the program and formulating new components based on current research and clinical practice. We are also grateful to Arthur Anastopoulos for his assistance as both a therapist and collaborator during the initial three years of this research program, and to Kenneth Fletcher for managing and analyzing our data sets.

We also wish to express our sincere appreciation to Seymour Weingarten and Robert Matloff of The Guilford Press for their receptiveness to the idea of this clinical manual and their willingness to undertake its publication. All of the authors are grateful to Anna Brackett for copyediting the book and overseeing its production. Russell Barkley continues to express his gratitude to his wife, Pat, and his children, Stephen and Kenneth, for their support of all of his writing endeavors. Gwen Edwards would like to thank the 70 families of oppositional ADHD teens who participated in our recent research project on family therapies for parent–teen conflict for their willingness to participate in that project and for all that they have taught her about parent–adolescent relations. And Arthur Robin wishes to express his appreciation to his wife, Susan, for her loving support of his scholarly pursuits. The wisdom we have all gained from the many and unique experiences each has had with our own teenagers is undoubtedly contained in the ideas expressed here.

# Contents

**Introduction**                                                                                     1

**Part I**  Prerequisite Information for Using the Program                                           15

**Chapter 1**  The Rationale for the Program                                                         17
**Chapter 2**  Clinical Assessment of Defiant Adolescents                                            44
**Chapter 3**  An Overview of the Family Training Program                                            72

**Part II**  Session Instructions                                                                    81

**Step 1**   Discussion of ADHD and ODD                                                              83
**Step 2**   Principles of Behavior Management                                                       87
**Step 3**   Developing Positive Attention                                                           95
**Step 4**   Developing Parental Attending Skills                                                   100
**Step 5**   Establishing a Behavioral Contract                                                     104
**Step 6**   Using Response Cost                                                                     109
**Step 7**   Completing the Contract/Point System                                                   113
**Step 8**   Grounding                                                                               116
**Step 9**   School Advocacy                                                                         119
**Step 10**  Introduction to Problem-Solving Communication Training                                  125
**Step 11**  Practicing Problem Solving                                                              133
**Step 12**  Practicing Problem Solving, Continued                                                   136
**Step 13**  Introduction to Communication Skills                                                    139

**Step 14**  Practicing Communication Skills                                          143

**Step 15**  Dealing with Unreasonable Beliefs and Expectations                      145

**Step 16**  Practicing Problem-Solving and Communication Skills:                    150
            Catching Unreasonable Beliefs

**Step 17**  More Family Practice                                                    153

**Step 18**  Concluding Treatment                                                    155

**Part III**  Assessment Materials                                                   157

General Instructions for Completing the Questionnaires (Form 1)                       160

Child and Family Information Form (Form 2)                                            162

Developmental and Medical History Form (Form 3)                                       163

Disruptive Behavior Disorders Rating Scale—Parent Form (Form 4)                       166

Disruptive Behavior Disorders Rating Scale—Teacher Form (Form 5)                      168

Clinical Interview—Parent Report Form (Form 6)                                        169

Adult Behavior Rating Scale—Self-Report of Current Behavior (Form 7)                  194

Adult Behavior Rating Scale—Self-Report of Childhood Behavior (Form 8)                195

Issues Checklist for Parents and Teenagers (Form 9)                                   196

**Part IV**  Parent Handouts for Steps 1–18                                          199

Parent Handout for Step 2:    Principles of Behavior Management                       203

Parent Handout for Step 2:    Coercive Behavior Cycle                                 204

Parent Handout for Step 3:    Paying Attention to Your Teen's Good Behavior           205

Parent Handout for Step 4:    How to Give Effective Commands                          207

Parent Handout for Step 5:    Sample Behavioral Contract                              208

Parent Handout for Step 5:    The Home Point System                                   210

Parent Handout for Step 8:    Grounding                                              211

Parent Handout for Step 9:    Accommodations for Improving Teen                       212
                              School Performance

Parent Handout for Step 9:    1991 Memorandum from the U.S. Department                213
                              of Education

Parent Handout for Step 10:   Steps to Better Problem Solving                         219

Parent Handout for Step 10:   Problem-Solving Worksheet                               220

Parent Handout for Step 10:   Problem-Solving Exercise                                221

Parent Handout for Step 13:   Communication Habits                     225

Parent Handout for Step 15:   Unreasonable Beliefs Chart              226

Adolescent Handout for Step 15:   Unreasonable Beliefs Chart       230


**References**                                                                                  233

**Index**                                                                                          246

# Introduction

## Purposes of Program

As with Barkley's earlier clinical manual for training parents of defiant children (Barkley, 1987, 1997), this manual is designed to serve several purposes. First, it provides a summary of clinical research on the nature of Oppositional Defiant Disorder (ODD) in children and adolescents, a condition with which Attention-Deficit/Hyperactivity Disorder (ADHD) is often a comorbid disorder. Second, it sets forth detailed instructions for conducting clinical evaluations of defiant or behavior-problem teenagers. Interview forms and behavior rating scales for conducting such evaluations are also provided here. These forms may be photocopied, as necessary, with permission of the publisher for use by the clinician in his or her own clinical practice. Some forms are also designed to be used for the periodic evaluation of the family and their response to the treatment program. Third, and more to the point, the manual specifies step-by-step procedures for conducting an effective, empirically validated program to train parents in the management of behavior-problem teens and train both parents and adolescents in effective problem-solving skills and communication styles. The format for the presentation of each step of the program has been carefully prepared so that the manual can be of utmost practical use, and the manual itself has been given a comb-binding so that it can lay flat on a desk or clipboard for easy reference during training sessions. Finally, this manual provides a set of family handouts to be used during the course of the program. These handouts include forms to be completed by the family members as well as instructions for the parent to use with each session of the program. The handouts are designed to be easy to read and brief in content. They are not meant to be used, however, in isolation, without training by a skilled child or family therapist.

It is critically important that the user of this manual and of the program it describes understand that this program is not intended for use by individuals who have not had the education and training necessary to provide mental health services to behavior problem adolescents and their families. Professionals using this program should have sound training in child development, child psychopathology, social-learning and behavior-modification techniques, family therapy, and/or other clinical interventions with families. In short, this program is not a substitute for the clinical training required for its implementation nor for the careful exercise of clinical judgment and ethics in dealing with behavior-problem teens and their families. The utmost care is always required in individually tailoring these methods to the particular characteristics of a given adolescent and his or her family.

We do not intend this manual to be a review of the scientific literature on parent training, family therapy programs, or research on defiant adolescents. Reviews of this literature as well as other approaches to family training have been published in numerous forums (see Loeber, 1990; Mash & Barkley, 1996, 1998; Patterson, 1982; Patterson, Reid, & Dishion, 1992; Robin & Foster, 1989). The reader may wish to consult these and other sources before undertaking this particular treatment approach. Instead we intended for this manual to serve as a clinical handbook for conducting only those procedures pertinent to this particular sequence of family training methods.

## Adolescents and Families Who May Be Appropriate Candidates for This Program

As with any clinical procedure, this program was not designed as a blanket method nor panacea to be applied to all teens and their families regardless of the family's presenting problems. It is expressly intended for teenagers who display noncompliant, defiant, oppositional, stubborn, or socially hostile behavior toward their parents either alone or in conjunction with other disorders. These teens are often referred to as having "externalizing" or "acting out" disorders and may be given the more generic layman's labels of difficult, defiant, or aggressive children, or the more specific clinical diagnoses of ODD, ADHD, Conduct Disorder (CD), or even juvenile-onset Bipolar Disorder, provided that noncompliant or defiant behavior is a primary problem. The program is also quite applicable to adolescents with mild developmental delay (mental retardation) where noncompliance or defiance is a problem in parent–teen interactions. Despite being intended for use with clinically referred populations of adolescents, however, portions of the program also may be quite valuable for use with mild situational family conflicts or behavior problems in otherwise normal teens whose families are being seen for more general parental, marital, or family therapy. In particular, teens displaying difficult, "acting out," or defiant behaviors as part of adjustment reactions to parental separation or divorce often respond well to the methods in this program. In short, when listening to and complying with parental commands or requests or adhering to household or neighborhood rules is problematic for an adolescent, this program may prove quite useful.

The program was designed for teens whose language level, general cognitive developmental level, or mental age is that of a 10-year-old or higher and whose chronological age falls between 13 and 18 years of age. While the parent training skills taught in Sessions 1–9 can be used with younger children, it would be preferable to follow the guidelines of the original program for children developed by Barkley (1997) and published elsewhere. It is our opinion that the problem-solving communication training (PSCT) elements of this program require a child be at least 13–14 years of age before undertaking those sessions (10–18) that require adolescent involvement in the problem-focused discussions.

The program has been successfully employed with single-parent as well as two-parent families, those of low income or educational levels, and even abusive families, although again the constraints and intended audience of this manual noted above apply here as well. Even when the teen in an abusive family is compliant, this program can serve to provide parents with more humane and effective methods of dealing with the everyday management of such a teen.

The program can certainly stand alone, and often does, as the primary form of intervention provided to parents of defiant teens. However, it can also serve as an adjunct to other forms of therapy being provided to troubled parents or families who also happen to have misbehaving adolescents. Many therapists have found a behavioral family training program such as this to be highly useful as an adjunct to marital counseling, when disagreements over teen management are an issue in the marriage (see Sanders, 1996, for a discussion of this issue with behavior-problem children), or to psychotherapy with anxious, depressed, or otherwise maladjusted adults who are also having problems managing the behavior of their teens. The program can also serve as part of a larger treatment package for socially aggressive, oppositional, or conduct-problem adolescents, who may themselves benefit from the addition of direct family training in social problem-solving skills (Kazdin, Esveldt-Dawson, French, & Unis, 1987; Kazdin, Siedel, & Bass, 1992).

Adolescents who are seriously aggressive and assaultive with others should not be considered candidates for this program. They often do not respond well, and their reaction to the procedures may result in an escalation of family conflicts. In rare instances, an increase in the adolescent's already destructive, verbally aggressive, or even physically assaultive behavior can occur when parents attempt some limit-setting on teen behavior, creating even more distress for the family than existed prior to treatment (Barkley et al., 1992).

Severely aggressive and defiant teenagers may be better treated with more intensive and multiple in-clinic therapies (Patterson, Dishion, & Chamberlain, 1993), in-home multisystemic forms of therapy (Mann, Borduin, Hengeler, & Blaske, 1990), or within-treatment foster care, day hospital programs, residential treatment facilities or inpatient child psychiatry units. At the conclusion of such interventions, parents and teens then can be trained in the procedures in this manual to prepare them for the adolescent's return to the home.

## Goals of the Program

The present program has a limited number of goals but is effective at achieving them with many families. They are as follows:

1. To improve parental management skills and competence in dealing with teen behavior problems, particularly noncompliant or defiant behavior.

2. To increase parental knowledge of the causes of defiant behavior in adolescents and the principles and concepts underlying the social learning of such behavior.

3. To improve teen cooperation with parental requests, directives, and rules.

4. To increase family harmony through the improvement of parental use of positive attention and other consequences with their teens, the provision of clear guidance, rules, and instruction to those teens, the application of swift, fair, and just discipline for inappropriate teen behavior, and the reliance on principle-guided parenting behavior more generally.

5. To increase both parental and teen use of problem-solving skills and positive communication styles during problem-focused discussions and interactions that involve the teen.

6. To alter the teen's or the parents' unreasonable beliefs, should they be observed to be guiding either parent or teen behavior during parent–teen problem-focused interactions.

## Outcomes Expected from This Program

The procedures described in Steps 1–9 here have a substantial amount of research supporting their efficacy with children up to approximately age 12 years of age (Anastopoulos, Shelton, DuPaul, & Guevremont, 1993; Forehand & McMahon, 1981; McMahon & Forehand, 1984; Patterson, 1982; Patterson, Dishion, & Chamberlain, 1993; Patterson et al., 1992; Sanders, 1996; Webster-Stratton, 1982; Webster-Stratton & Spitzer, 1996). Each procedure is supported by published studies demonstrating significant improvements in child behavior as a function of these or highly similar behavior management methods, including (1) *improving parental selective attending skills* (Eyberg & Robinson, 1982; Forehand & McMahon, 1981; Kelley, Embry, & Baer, 1979; Patterson, 1982; Pollard, Ward, & Barkley, 1983; Pisterman et al., 1989; Roberts, 1985; Webster-Stratton, Hollinsworth, & Kolpacoff, 1989); (2) *improving parental deliverance of requests* (Blum, Williams, Friman, & Christophersen, 1995; Forehand & McMahon, 1981; Green, Forehand, & McMahon, 1979; Patterson, 1982; Roberts, McMahon, Forehand, & Humphreys, 1978; Williams & Forehand, 1984); (3) *improving children's independent play behavior* (Anastopoulos et al., 1993; Pollard et al., 1983; Wahler & Fox, 1980); (4) *parental use of time out as a disciplinary method* (Anastopoulos et al., 1993; Bean & Roberts, 1981; Day & Roberts, 1982; Eyberg & Robinson, 1982; Forehand & McMahon, 1981; Patterson, 1982; Pisterman et al., 1989; Roberts et al., 1979; Roberts, Hatzenbuehler, & Bean, 1981; Strayhorn & Weidman, 1989; Wahler & Fox, 1980; Webster-Stratton et al., 1989); (5) *parental use of response cost as a disciplinary method* (Anastopoulos et al., 1993; Little & Kelley, 1989); and (6) *parental planning and activity scheduling as problem-prevention measures*, particularly before entering public places (Anastopoulos et al., 1993; Pisterman et al., 1989; Sanders & Christensen, 1984; Sanders & Dadds, 1982; Sanders & Glynn, 1981).

Typically, up to 64% or more of the families of defiant children undergoing training in such methods report significant improvement in their children's behavior and their own parenting abilities. Yet research also suggests that when used alone with older adolescents who have ODD (or ADHD), the behavioral parent training program benefits only about 25% of families, while 35% or so benefit from the separate PSCT component (Barkley, Guevremont, Anastopoulos, & Fletcher, 1992). Although such results may seem disappointing at first blush, more traditional family therapy programs may produce even fewer positive responders to treatment, on the order of just 10% in one of our earlier projects (Barkley, Guevremont, et al., 1992). Moreover, research suggests that many forms of parent and family training appear to decline in their efficacy (as determined by percentage of families responding to treatment) as the age group of children targeted in such programs changes to adolescence (Dishion & Patterson, 1992). It is also our belief that combinations of earlier programs are needed to address the more long-lasting and intransigent defiant behavior of adolescents with ODD (and often ADHD), which is why we have combined behavioral parent training with the PSCT program and extended therapy from 9 to 18 sessions. Evidence arising from our ongoing NIMH-funded family training research project clearly suggests that the combination of these two programs is superior to either of them used alone, especially in reducing drop-out rates.

These declines in the effectiveness of family-focused interventions with clinic-referred defiant adolescents in comparison to the similar treatment of clinic-referred defiant children may also be the result of another process rarely discussed in the family therapy literature. That process is the increasing contribution of genetic influences to parent–child conflict and the child's antisocial behavior as the age of the child increases. That is, research seems to suggest that within-family social influences on child misbehavior may be greater during early childhood, diminishing with the age of the child (Rowe, 1994). In contrast, the genetic contribution to individual differences in antisocial behavior and parent–teen conflict increases with age (Braungart-Reiker, Rende, Plomin, DeFries, & Fulker, 1995; Elkins, McGue, & Iacono, 1997; Pike, McGuire, Hetherington, Reiss, & Plomin, 1996; Pike, Reiss, Hetherington, & Plomin, 1996). In short, genetic factors account for most of the variance in parent–teen conflict and teen antisocial behavior at late adolescence. How can this be? Perhaps it is as Scarr and McCartney (1983) have suggested: older children have more choice in the kinds of environments they create for themselves and in the involvement or relationships they are likely to have with their parents. This has been called "niche-picking" (Scarr & McCartney, 1983; Scarr, 1992) or "the extended phenotype" (Dawkins, 1982). It refers to the likelihood that individuals with given genotypes not only increasingly choose the kinds of environments in which to live but increasingly construct such environments around themselves such that gene–environment interactions increase with age. The environments and relationships in which they are found, then, increasingly reflect aspects of their own phenotype, or extensions of their genotype futher into their environmental ecologies. With increasing age, then, children are likely to exert increasing influence on their environment and to be less affected by the environment themselves. Individual differences in both behavior toward and relationships with parents in adolescence may therefore be reflective more of child effects on adults than of adult effects on children. They may also be the result of shared genetic risk for comparable forms of psychopathology that increase risk for conflict. Thus, to the extent that such differences in child behavior and personality are genetically influenced, and many are (Rowe, 1994), those genetic influences will explain a greater proportion of the variance in conflicts and relations with parents at adolescence than they did earlier in life.

The net result of these processes for clinicians working with clinic-referred adolescents is that clinic-referred adolescents are likely to be considerably more difficult to treat successfully. Adolescent ODD, antisocial conduct, and negativity in parent–teen interactions may be far more influenced by genetic factors than by environmental ones, at least more so than are similar problems in younger clinic-referred children, who are much more responsive to parent training interventions. This is not to argue that biology is destiny or that such conflicts are therefore immutable; that would be a mistaken interpretation of the meaning of heritability in research on this issue. It is to say that such studies suggest that the shared environment (rearing environment) may not make as much a contribution to parent–teen conflict as does genetics, and so if the intent of family therapy is to address the root cause of such conflict, it is not likely to do so with great success. This suggests that clinicians might need to be content with a far lower success rates in their adolescent cases of ODD and CD than would be acceptable in child cases; therefore, response rates of 35% or more may be cause for optimism rather than pessimism.

As with any psychosocial program for families, the degree of success is greatly affected by the extent, nature, and severity of the teen's psychopathology, the psychopathology of the family, and other factors (see "Predictors of Success and Failure," below). With adolescents whose major problem is noncompliance or oppositional behavior and whose families are not seriously dysfunctional, this program usually results in the teen's behavior and compliance being brought within the range considered normal for that teen's age group. In our experience, teenagers with more serious forms of developmental psychopathology that are chronic in nature, such as ADHD, ODD, CD, Atypical Pervasive Developmental Disorder, or their combinations, may have improved interactions with their parents under this program. Nevertheless, even after treatment, many teens may continue to be rated more deviant in inattentive and impulsive behavior than normal children on behavior rating scales, particularly if the teens had significant degrees of symptoms of ADHD before treatment (Barkley, Guevremont, et al., 1992). This same phenomenon has also been observed in studies of parent training with ADHD children (Anastopoulos et al., 1993; Johnston, 1992). With such cases, our recommended attitude is one of training families to "cope" with the teen's problems rather than "cure" them; nevertheless, the program can reduce the extent to which noncompliance or defiance contributes to the teen's various problems and the distress within the family.

Older clinic-referred adolescents may benefit less than young adolescents from parent training programs, although some benefits still accrue to them and their families (Barkley et al., 1992; Dishion & Patterson, 1992). Older teens referred to clinics for treatment probably have had more years of effectively utilizing coercive behavior, especially that involving physical as well as verbal resistance; may have more severe defiant and conduct problems; may have more frank psychiatric disturbance; and may come from more disrupted or impaired families (Dishion & Patterson, 1992; Patterson et al., 1992).

Although we have no scientific data available as yet to support this view, it is our opinion that adolescents with ODD or CD who have comorbid ADHD are likely to respond much more positively to the program presented here if those teens are on stimulant medication for the management of their ADHD. Those medications result in a substantial reduction in impulsive, inattentive, and hyperactive behaviors, which can adversely affect both parent–teen interactions and general social and academic success. These medications have also been found to reduce levels of emotional, aggressive, and oppositional behavior, and even antisocial acts by such teens (DuPaul, Barkley, & Connor, 1998). For these reasons, we believe that adjunct stimulant medication may make such adolescents more amenable to and cooperative with the family training recommended in this manual.

Parents with at least a high school education and with a minimal degree of personal or family distress are likely to do quite well in acquiring and utilizing the skills and knowledge taught in this program. Such parents are also more likely to report high levels of consumer satisfaction with the training procedures (Calvert & McMahon, 1987; Forehand & McMahon, 1981; McMahon & Forehand, 1984; Patterson, 1982; Robin & Foster, 1989; Sanders, 1996; Webster-Stratton & Spitzer, 1996).

Studies have indicated that the methods of parent training in this program receive high ratings of social acceptability when reviewed by other adults or by the parents who are the direct recipients of the training (Calvert & McMahon, 1987; Kazdin, 1980; Sanders, 1996; Webster-Stratton & Spitzer, 1996). Such parents not only reported improved child behavior (Anastopoulos et al., 1993; Bernal, Klinnert, & Schultz, 1980; Dubey, O'Leary, & Kaufman, 1983; Eyberg & Robinson, 1982; Forehand & McMahon, 1981; Patterson, Chamberlain, & Reid, 1982; Pisterman et al., 1989; Pollard et al., 1983), but also demonstrated changes in directly observed parental behavior (Patterson, 1982; Patterson et al., 1982) and better attitudes toward their children (Forehand & McMahon, 1981; McMahon & Forehand, 1984; Webster-Stratton et al., 1989). Parents trained in behavior-management skills also reported increased knowledge of parenting skills, reduced parenting stress, improved self-esteem and parenting competence (Anastopoulos et al., 1992; Spaccarelli, Cotler, & Penman, 1992; Spitzer, Webster-Stratton, & Hollinsworth, 1991), better sibling behavior (Eyberg & Robinson, 1982; Humphreys, Forehand, McMahon, & Roberts, 1978), and better marital and family functioning (Forehand & McMahon, 1981).

Substantially less research has been done on this program or others like it with adolescents who have ODD, so it is unclear whether the same types and degrees of improvement can be expected with them. However, what research exists suggests that behavioral parent training programs as well as programs using approaches similar to PSCT do produce significant treatment effects on parent and teen functioning (Barkley, Guevremont, et al., 1992; Dishion & Andrews, 1995; Robin, 1981; Robin & Foster, 1989).

## Maintenance of Treatment Gains over Time

A number of studies of children with defiant behavior or ODD have examined the extent to which parents and children continue to manifest improved interactions with each other once treatment has been terminated. Improvement in child behavior, parent behavior, and parental attitudes toward their children have all been found to be maintained over periods of 3 months to 4.5 years and even 9 to 14 years after treatment termination (see Estrada & Pinsof, 1995, for a review; Dubey et al., 1983; Forehand & McMahon, 1981; McMahon & Forehand, 1984; Patterson, 1982; Patterson & Fleischman, 1979; Patterson et al., 1992; Pisterman et al., 1989; Strain, Steele, Ellis, & Timm, 1982; Webster-Stratton, 1982; Webster-Stratton et al., 1989). Yet several studies have noted that parental use of positive attending skills to prosocial child behavior are less likely to be maintained at follow-up than are the parents' use of other skills taught in the program (Patterson, 1982; Webster-Stratton, 1982; Webster-Stratton et al., 1989). Despite this decline in parental positive attending skills after treatment termination, gains in child behavior found at the end of treatment continue to be maintained across follow-up periods up to 4.5 years later. This wealth of studies reflecting the maintenance of treatment gains over time is encouraging, but it is not found in all research studies of parent training. A few studies have not found long-term effects of behavioral parent training (Bernal et al., 1980; Strayhorn & Weidman, 1991), suggesting that lasting gains are not always the norm for all forms of behavioral parent training.

Once again, we must note that research on the use of behavioral parent training with teenagers who have defiant behavior or ODD is far less substantial than with children, and thus it is not clear to what extent gains produced by family-based training programs such as this one are maintained over time after termination. We are examining this issue in our own ongoing research with this program, in which parents and teens are reevaluated several months after treatment termination. Encouraging findings of maintenance of treatment effects over a 10-week follow-up period have been reported for families undergoing the PSCT component of this program (Robin, 1981). Dishion and Andrews (1995) have also reported results for a behavioral parent training program for adolescents similar to this one in which reductions in behavioral problems (as reported by parents) achieved by the treatment program were maintained for up to 1 year after treatment termination. Important to note in that study was the finding that treatments that focused only on teens in groups actually resulted in an increase in both problem behaviors and tobacco smoking by 1-year follow-up. Such findings argue for the inclusion of parent-focused treatment efforts in dealing with behavior-problem teens. Certainly the issue of maintenance of treatment gains from family training with adolescents who have ODD is a most important one and is deserving of far greater research than has been the case to date.

## Generalization of Treatment Gains across Settings

Therapists as well as school staff may be tempted to believe that parental participation in behavioral parent training programs at the offices of mental health professionals or even in the parents' homes will result in improved teen behavior at school. Unfortunately, most studies of behavior-problem children have not found such generalization of treatment gains to school settings to occur (Horn, Ialongo, Greenberg, Packard, & Smith-Winberry, 1990; Horn, Ialongo, Popovich, & Peradotto, 1987; McMahon & Forehand, 1984; Patterson, 1982), although at least one has done so (Strayhorn & Weidman, 1991). Some studies have found that children whose parents received parent training, or at least a subset of such children, manifest improved school conduct, but that just as many children within those studies either showed no change in school behavior or a significant worsening of such behavior (Firestone, Kelly, Goodman, & Davey, 1981; McMahon & Forehand, 1984). None of the studies that failed to find generalization of treatment effects to school settings, however, directly targeted school behavior problems as part of the parent training program. Consequently, therapists using traditional behavioral parent training programs should not encourage either parents or school staff to believe that generalization of gains to child school behavior is likely to occur. This was one of the reasons why we have added a session to the original version of Barkley's program to help parents assist teachers with improving their child's school conduct and performance through the use of home-based reward programs and homework goal-setting procedures. Such procedures have been shown to result in improved teacher ratings of school behavior and improved homework performance (Atkeson & Forehand, 1978; Kelley, 1990).

In the case of clinic-referred adolescents undergoing similar types of parent and family training, far less research exists on the issue of generalization of treatment effects. Dishion and Andrews (1995) found only a marginally significant immediate treatment effect of parent training on teen school behavior problems (as rated by teachers). And this effect dissipated to some degree over the 1-year follow-up period. Thus it seems wise to continue to counsel families that parent/family training programs with teens, as with children, are unlikely to result in automatic improvements in school conduct and performance in the absence of specific treatment methods designed to promote such generalization.

## Predictors of Success and Failure

Research with the behavioral parent training program (Steps 1–9) suggests that up to 64% or more of families with ADHD and/or clinically serious oppositional children may expect clinically significant change or recovery (normalization) as a result of this program (Anastopoulos et al., 1993; Pisterman et al., 1989; Quici, Wheeler, & Bolle, 1996) and similar such programs (Bernal et al., 1980; Dishion & Patterson, 1992; Webster-Stratton et al., 1989). The percentage improved is greater among younger (<6 years) and less clinically severe children than among older children or adolescents (Dishion &

Patterson, 1992; Webster-Stratton et al., 1989). But not all families can be expected to benefit from a behavioral parent training program such as this one. Research on similar such programs suggests a number of factors that are related to program ineffectiveness when programs were used with children: number of sessions attended, failure to complete training or return for follow-up, reduced level of improvement in parent and child conflicts. There is no reason to believe similar factors would not emerge as moderators of treatment success with adolescents. Such factors should be considered by therapists as a possible basis on which to assign families to group parent training (good likelihood of responding) versus individual training (higher number of risk factors) or to offer parent training versus other, more parent-focused treatments (Holden, Lavigne, & Cameron, 1990).

## Child Factors

Only a few child characteristics have been identified as related to the effectiveness of behavioral parent training programs. As noted above, one relatively consistent predictor of diminished effectiveness of parent training is the age of the child. Preschool children (<6 years old) appear to have the highest rates of positive responding to behavioral parent training programs (65% or more); school-age children are somewhat less likely to improve (50–64%) (Anastopoulos et al., 1993; Dishion & Patterson, 1992; Strain et al., 1982; Strain, Young, & Horowitz, 1981); and adolescents are the least likely (25–35%; Barkley, Guevremont, et al., 1992). However, this effect of age actually might be an inverted U-shaped or curvilinear function, in that within the preschool-age group, higher parental drop-out rates and lower degrees of responding have been found to be associated with *younger* ages of the children (Holden et al., 1990). And even within the elementary age range, the effect of age on treatment responding has been found to be the opposite of that noted above, with parents of younger children more likely to discontinue treatment prematurely (Firestone & Witt, 1982). Higher intelligence or mental age in children has also been associated positively with better response to parent training or parental persistence through a parent training program (Firestone & Witt, 1982).

The severity of the child's behavioral problems, and defiance specifically, has been noted in some studies as being correlated with more limited treatment efficacy and a greater likelihood of parental premature termination from training (Dumas, 1984; Holden et al., 1990). But this relationship might be explained by another one, that being the relationship of parental stress, marital distress, and parental psychopathology to the severity of the child's problems (Webster-Stratton & Hammond, 1990). That is, the severity of the child's problems simply serves as a marker for more important parent factors (see section below), which cause parents to terminate training prematurely or to fail to respond positively to the training. In our earlier study of behavioral parent training with families in which there are ODD/ADHD adolescents, we were unable to identify pretreatment variables that significantly predicted the degree of change that occurred during treatment (Barkley, Guevremont, et al., 1992).

As noted above, adolescents with ADHD who are also defiant and whose parents undergo this training program should not be expected to be "recovered" or normalized in all of their behavioral problems as a consequence of this program. Research with both children and adolescents suggests that defiant and hostile behavior is likely to improve the most from this program, and ADHD symptoms are likely to improve only somewhat or not at all (Anastopoulos et al., 1993; Barkley, Guevremont, et al., 1992; Johnston, 1992). Thus, stimulant medication or other pharmacological therapy may need to be added to the treatment package provided to such children in order to better address comorbid ADHD (Firestone et al., 1981).

Where stimulant medication is used, therapists may find that there is sometimes little additional benefit provided to families by the addition of a parent training program, as was found in some studies of ADHD children (Abikoff & Hechtman, 1995; Firestone et al., 1981; Horn et al., 1991). Given that stimulant medications have proven to be among the most effective treatments for children and adolescents with ADHD (DuPaul et al., 1998; Rapport & Kelly, 1993; Swanson, McBurnett, Christian, & Wigal, 1995), we have amended the training program to suggest a discussion of this issue for parents of ADHD teens in the initial session of the program when the subject of ADHD arises. Therapists wishing more information about psychopharmacology for ADHD children and teens are referred to the texts by Werry and Aman (1998), Weiss (1992), Greenhill and Osman (1991), and the spring 1990 issue of the *Journal of Child and Adolescent Psychopharmacology* (Vol. 1, Issue 1).

## Parent Factors

Research on behavioral parent training for child behavior problems finds that parents who are relatively younger than the average of those seeking training, are less intelligent, have less than a high school education, and are in a lower social class usually do not achieve the same degree of success as do others (Dumas, 1984; Firestone & Witt, 1982; Holden et al., 1990; Knapp & Deluty, 1989; Webster-Stratton & Hammond, 1990). However, the detrimental effects of lower socioeconomic status have not always been noted in studies of behavioral parent training with children (McMahon & Forehand, 1984; Rogers, Forehand, Griest, Wells, & McMahon, 1981). One study also found that family ethnic group was associated with dropping out of treatment or progressing more slowly through training, with minority groups having more of these difficulties than the majority group (Holden et al., 1990). However, social class was also found to show the same relationship to poor progress through treatment, and it, rather than ethnic group, may actually have created this difference given the differential representation of such groups across social class. As might be expected, the number of required sessions the parents' actually attended in the training program has been shown to be related to treatment efficacy (Strain et al., 1981). Whether or not such parent factors are associated with success in family treatments focusing on adolescents with behavior problems is uncertain given the relatively limited research examining this issue with teens in treatment.

Diminished benefits from parent training and even higher drop-out rates from training are especially likely for parents (mothers) who are socially isolated from adult peers in their community and who encounter aversive interactions with their extended family, according to research on conduct-problem children (Dumas, 1984; Dumas & Wahler, 1983; Salzinger, Kaplan, & Artemyeff, 1983; Wahler, 1980; Wahler & Afton, 1980). Even when such parents demonstrate improved child management and fewer parent–child conflicts, they may have a greater likelihood of relapse after training concludes (Dumas & Wahler, 1983; Wahler, 1980; Wahler & Afton, 1980). Dumas and Wahler (1983) have shown that maternal insularity (isolation) when combined with socioeconomic disadvantage accounted for nearly 50% of the variance in treatment effectiveness, suggesting that these may be two of the most important factors in assessing the likelihood that a family will respond positively to behavioral parent training. It is possible, however, that if there is greater involvement and training from the therapist as well as more time for practice (Knapp & Deluty, 1989), and if the therapist addresses the mothers' social isolation before undertaking training or during training (Dadds & McHugh, 1992; Dumas & Wahler, 1983; Wahler, Cartor, Fleischman, & Lambert, 1993), these families might be able achieve significant improvements in child or teen management.

Parents with serious forms of psychopathology (psychosis, severe depression, alcohol/drug dependency, etc.), do not seem to do well in parent training programs such as this one, at least as it has been studied with conduct-problem children (Patterson & Chamberlain, 1992). Those parents start out resistant to training and homework assignments and seem to remain so throughout treatment. Also, research on parent training with children shows that those parents demonstrating greater negativity and helplessness as well as those having poor anger control typically do not respond as positively in such training programs, or are more likely to drop out of treatment (Frankel & Simmons, 1992). Perhaps providing training in more effective general problem-solving skills (Pfiffner, Jouriles, Brown, Etscheidt, & Kelly, 1988; Prinz & Miller, 1994; Spaccarelli et al., 1992) or anger-management skills prior to or as an adjunct to parent training in child management may prove useful in enhancing the effectiveness of parent training programs (see Goldstein, Keller, & Erne, 1985, and Sanders, 1996, for a discussion). That is certainly the premise of the present hybrid family training program, in which different treatment approaches have been combined in an effort to enhance treatment efficacy.

One parent characteristic that will likely receive increased attention in research on parent training in the coming decade is the relationship of parental ADHD to child or teen ODD and to parental responsiveness to parent training. ADHD in children is known to have a strong hereditary predisposition (see Barkley, 1998, for discussion) with an average of 25% of immediately family members likely to have the disorder. This means that there is at least a 50% chance that one of the ADHD child's biological parents is an adult with ADHD. Up to 65% of children with ODD are likely to have ADHD as a comorbid disorder, and even those who do not are likely to be more difficult to manage than are normal children, making childhood ADHD highly likely among children whose families are recommended for behavioral parent training programs such as this one. This suggests that not only is there a significant probability that the child who is the focus of the parent training efforts has ADHD, but that one of the child's parents has ADHD as well. Evans, Vellano, and Pelham (1994) have discussed the detrimental effects parental ADHD may have on the parent training process and have even shown that treatment of parental ADHD with stimulant medication may prove useful in facilitating a positive response of that parent to the parent training course. For these reasons, assessment instruments have been included in this program to assist clinicians in screening for both the presence of adolescent ADHD as well as parental ADHD.

Past research with conduct-problem children suggests that the degree of marital discord is also a predictor of diminished effectiveness of parent training within this and other parent training programs (Forehand & McMahon, 1981; Patterson, 1982; Webster-Stratton & Hammond, 1990). Perhaps it is better to provide such parents with marital therapy (Dadds, Schwartz, & Sanders, 1987) or divorce counseling to help resolve their marital problems before parent training in child management is offered, or at least as an adjunct to it. As might be expected, whether or not the family was intact (parents married) at the time of training is also a predictor of responding to parent training programs, with single-parent families responding less well than two-parent households (Strain et al., 1981, 1982; Webster-Stratton & Hammond, 1990). Degree of life stress experienced within the past year may also be associated with reduced parent training efficacy (Webster-Stratton & Hammond, 1990). It is not clear as yet whether these same predictors would apply equally well to predicting response to family training programs involving conduct-problem teens, but there is little reason to believe that they would not apply.

## Therapist Factors

As discussed in an earlier text (Barkley, 1997), increasing attention has been paid to the role that therapist factors play in the success of behavioral parent training programs. Such factors long have been known to be of importance in studies of psychotherapy outcomes with adults (Garfield & Bergen, 1986) and, more recently, in psychotherapy studies with children (Crits-Christoph & Mintz, 1991; Kazdin, 1991). A few studies have examined this issue relative to behavioral parent training, particularly Patterson's research team at the Oregon Social Learning Center. Trainee therapists do not appear to be as effective in maintaining parents in parent training programs as are more experienced therapists (Frankel & Simmons, 1992). Moreover, among experienced therapists, those who tend to teach and confront parents are more likely to encounter parent resistance to training than are those who facilitate and support parents in the process of training (Patterson & Forgatch, 1985). Resistance in such families can occur within the session to the formal training procedures themselves as well as to the homework assignments parents are required to perform (Patterson & Chamberlain, 1992). Patterson and Chamberlain (1992) report that parent trainers working with families of seriously antisocial children can expect to encounter resistance from most families at the start of treatment, and that such resistance is likely to increase until the midpoint of treatment. In less serious cases and with parents of younger children, this resistance may be addressed and resolved by the therapist by treatment termination. In more difficult cases, resistance is likely to persist at high levels, foreboding fewer changes in parental management skills and an overall less positive outcome. Such client resistance is likely to provoke the therapist to confront behaviors, but this, as noted above, may increase client resistance. Thus, parent-training therapists must achieve a delicate balance between teaching and confronting parental resistance and providing facilitation and support to motivate the parents to undertake behavioral change (Patterson & Chamberlain, 1992). It has been our experience in working with families of clinic-referred conduct-problem teenagers that the issue of family resistance to change is even more applicable (and more frustrating to therapists!) than it might be in families of behavior-problem children.

## Organization of the Manual

Like its child-focused predecessor (Barkley, 1997), this training manual has been organized into three sections: Part I provides information on the background of this program, its theoretical and research basis, methods of evaluating oppositional and defiant children both before and after treatment, and various prerequisite information to consider before undertaking this program of therapy. As noted earlier, much of this information has been taken from the earlier manual on defiant children (Barkley, 1997) with modification, as appropriate, for an adolescent population. Part II provides detailed instructions on conducting each of the 18 steps of the program. Clinicians should acquaint themselves thoroughly with the steps and periodically review the contents of each one while training families. Each step in this section begins with the goals of that step followed by an outline of the material to be taught in that step such that a clinician experienced in this program need only refer to these outlines during training sessions with a family. Part III contains the assessment tools that are used during the pre- and posttreatment evaluation of the teenagers and their families as well as the handouts to be used with each step of the program.

## Summary

The procedures we have set forth in this manual are designed specifically for families with adolescents who are noncompliant, defiant, or oppositional and who range in age from 13 to 18 years. The methods are meant to be employed by experienced clinicians with adequate training in delivering psychological services to families of defiant adolescents. Although effective, the success of these procedures is dependent upon the nature and severity of the teen's problems, the teen's age, the extent and severity of parental and family psychopathology, and the level of parental intelligence and motivation to utilize these methods, among other factors. When taught properly, this program can be beneficial in diminishing or eliminating parent–adolescent conflict and behavior problems in teenagers.

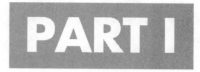

# Prerequisite Information for Using the Program

# CHAPTER 1

# The Rationale for the Program

In this chapter we discuss the primary emphasis of the family training program: teen oppositional defiant behavior and parent–teen conflict, or teen noncompliance. In so doing, we present the rationale behind selecting this focus and the results of research that buttress that focus. As in its counterpart manual for working with defiant children (Barkley, 1997b), we have selected this target for intervention because it can be clearly defined, has relevance to the presenting complaints of the teenager and family, is an important predictor of the teen's present and future adjustment, and is grounded in a scientific theory of its development and maintenance (Mash & Terdal, 1997).

## Noncompliance Defined

We employ the term "noncompliance" here to refer to three somewhat separate yet overlapping categories of teen conduct:

1. *Failure to initiate behaviors requested by an adult within a reasonable time after a directive has been given by that adult.* In most cases, *a reasonable time* refers to a minute or so after the command was given, although parents may specifically stipulate when compliance is to be initiated (e.g., "When that TV show is over, you are to clean-up your room."). Research on noncompliance has generally used a more stringent interval of 10–15 seconds after a command was given as a reasonable time for compliance to be initiated, but with teenagers we believe that a somewhat more liberal standard is typical of most families, comparable to a situation in which an adult might be given a similar request.

2. *Failure to sustain compliance to a directive until the requirements stipulated in that instruction have been fulfilled.* Some may consider this behavior category a form of sustained attention to tasks ("on task" behavior), or persistence of effort.

3. *Failure to follow previously taught rules of conduct in a situation.* Such behaviors as leaving the house without permission, stealing, lying, hitting or aggressing against others, taking food from the kitchen without permission, taking money from parents wallets without permission, and swearing at parents are just a few forms of teen conduct that parents would consider to be violations of previously taught standards of conduct.

Using the term "noncompliance" for these forms of misconduct conveys passive avoidance of parental instructions or household rules. The term "defiance" is best used for those instances when the teen manifests active verbal or physical resistance to cooperation with parental directives, as in the case of verbal refusal, temper outbursts, and even physically aggressing against a parent when compliance with a parental directive attempts to be imposed by the parent on the child. Some examples of noncompliant and defiant behaviors are shown in Table 1.1, though this list is hardly exhaustive. These behaviors belong to a general class of behavior that involves noncompliance, or what some have called hostile–defiant behavior or social aggression. Some of the behaviors in Table 1.1 are in fact direct efforts of the teen to escape or avoid the imposition of the directive (see Patterson, 1982; or Patterson et al., 1992). Hence, all of these forms of conduct may be treated in a single program that addresses noncompliance. Research, at least in elementary-age children, has shown that treating noncompliance often results in significant improvements in other behaviors in this general class even when those other behaviors were not specifically targeted by the intervention (Russo, Cataldo, & Cushing, 1981; Wells, Forehand, & Griest, 1980). It is this targeting of noncompliance and the parent–teen conflict that is invariably associated with it that distinguishes this family training program. Many other programs single out one or several types of inappropriate behavior for family therapy yet fail to address the more general class of noncompliance to which such specific forms of noncompliance and conflict belong.

Another means of understanding the relationships among various forms of disruptive behavior comes from meta-analytic reviews of the literature employing factor analysis to study the relationships among these various forms of misconduct (Frick et al., 1993). These re-

**TABLE 1.1.** Types of Noncompliant and Defiant Behaviors Common in Children and Adolescents Referred for Behavior Disorders

| | | |
|---|---|---|
| Yells | Steals | Physically resists |
| Whines | Lies | Destroys property |
| Complains | Argues | Physically fights with others |
| Defies | Humiliates/annoys | Fails to complete school homework |
| Screams | Teases | Disrupts others' activities |
| Tantrums | Ignores requests | Ignores self-care tasks |
| Throws objects | Runs away | Sasses or talks back |
| Insults | Cries | |
| Swears | Fails to complete routine chores | |

*Note.* Adapted from Barkley (1997b, p. 18). Copyright 1997 by The Guilford Press. Adapted by permission.

lationships can best be captured in a two-dimensional grid (Figure 1.1), with the dimensions of Overt–Covert types of misconduct appearing orthogonal to that of Nondestructive–Destructive forms of misconduct. This figure demonstrates how the various forms of oppositional defiant behavior cluster into a nondestructive form of overt disruptive behavior that is related to three other equally if not more serious forms of antisocial acts, such as status violations and aggresion toward and offenses against others. Such a diagram implies that one could classify defiant teens into four somewhat separable groups based on this two-dimensional system. This study and others have shown that there is a developmental pattern to the staging of these subgroups, thereby underscoring the point that teen oppositional behavior and parent–teen conflict carry with them significant developmental risks for the progression of the teenager into more serious forms of conduct disorder, antisocial behavior, and even criminal activity (Lahey, Loeber, Quay, Frick, & Grimm, 1992; Lahey & Loeber, 1994; Loeber, 1988, 1990).

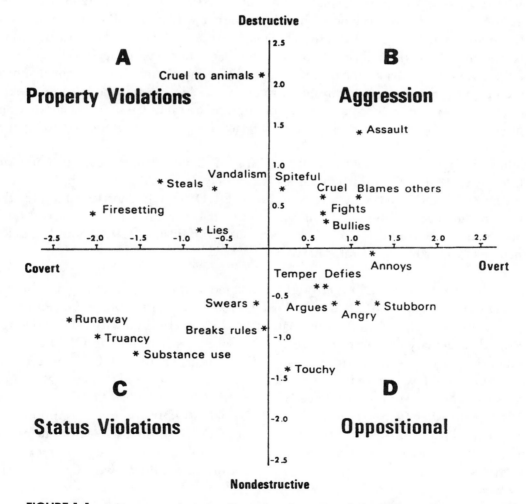

**FIGURE 1.1.** A diagram representing the results of a meta-analysis of factor analytic studies of disruptive child behavior. From Frick et al. (1993, p. 327). Copyright 1993 by Pergamon Press. Reprinted by permission.

## The Continuum of Teen Noncompliance/Defiance and Family Conflict

Noncompliant behavior can be thought of as representing a continuum or a dimension of conduct, the terms for which do not have a consensus of professional opinion. Adolescents whose defiant behavior is above the mean but within at least a single standard deviation (+1 *SD*) above the mean (approximately 84th percentile) on a well-standardized behavior rating scale of this dimension should be considered to fall within the normal range, even though they may be viewed as being stubborn, strong-willed, or firmly opinionated at times. Teens placing above the 84th percentile but below the 93rd percentile (within +1 to +1.5 *SDs*) could be described as being "noncompliant," as they would have been in childhood (Forehand & McMahon, 1981); as being "difficult to manage"; or as having borderline ODD. The latter is appropriate, of course, only in so far as the teen does not meet the full clinical diagnostic criteria for that disorder in the most recent *Diagnostic and Statistical Manual of Mental Disorders* (DSM-IV; American Psychiatric Association [APA], 1994). Those adolescents who place above the 93rd percentile on such rating scales or who meet full clinical criteria for ODD should be labelled with that disorder. This diagnosis could be further qualified by the prefixes of "mild," "moderate," or "severe," depending on the degree of deviance in ratings of defiant/oppositional behavior or on the number of ODD symptoms above the minimal number required to meet the diagnostic threshold. In our view, adolescents who fall into most of these categories except the normal one may be appropriate candidates for this family training program, as long as the conditions described later for justifying intervention were met.

The clinical diagnostic criteria from DSM-IV for ODD and its more severe counterpart, CD (see APA, 1994), are set forth in Tables 1.2 and 1.3. Bear in mind that the majority of adolescents with ODD and CD have comorbid ADHD. The diagnostic criteria for that disorder are provided in Table 1.4. Clinicians wishing to become more familiar with ADHD and its treatment will find the text by Barkley (1998), Hinshaw (1994), and Weiss and Hechtman (1993) to be quite informative.

Research has found that ODD is strongly associated with later risk for eventual childhood CD (Lahey et al., 1992; Lahey & Loeber, 1994; Loeber, 1998, 1990; Patterson, 1982; Patterson et al., 1992). Approximately 20–25% of children with ODD no longer have the disorder 3 years later. Yet up to 52% will persist in having ODD over this period of time. Among those with persistent ODD, nearly half (25% of the initial total of those with ODD) will have CD within a 3-year follow-up period (Lahey et al., 1992). Conversely, among children who have CD, over 80% will have had ODD as a prior or preexisting disorder (Lahey et al., 1992). This makes ODD the most common early developmental stage for the later progression into CD. To summarize, while the majority of ODD children will not progress further into CD, children with persistent ODD are more likely to do so. In addition, the vast majority of children with CD will arrive at CD by way of earlier ODD.

Other developmental pathways leading to CD also exist. These variations are apparently related to a subtype of later CD likely to emerge over time (Lahey & Loeber, 1994; Loeber,

**TABLE 1.2.** Diagnostic Criteria for Oppositional Defiant Disorder

A. A pattern of negativistic, hostile, and defiant behavior lasting at least 6 months, during which four (or more) of the following are present:

    (1) often loses temper
    (2) often argues with adults
    (3) often actively defies or refuses to comply with adults' requests or rules
    (4) often deliberately annoys people
    (5) often blames others for his or her mistakes or misbehavior
    (6) is often touchy or easily annoyed by others
    (7) is often angry and resentful
    (8) is often spiteful or vindictive

    **Note:** Consider a criterion met only if the behavior occurs more frequently than is typically observed in individuals of comparable age and developmental level.

B. The disturbance in behavior causes clinically significant impairment in social, academic, or occupational functioning.

C. The behaviors do not occur exclusively during the course of a Psychotic or Mood Disorder.

D. Criteria are not met for Conduct Disorder, and, if the individual is age 18 years or older, criteria are not met for Antisocial Personality Disorder.

*Note.* From American Psychiatric Association (1994, pp. 93–94). Copyright 1994 by the American Psychiatric Association. Reprinted by permission.

1988, 1990; Loeber et al., 1993; Patterson et al., 1992). A particularly important predictor of the progression into delinquency and the severity and persistence of such delinquency is the age of onset of early CD symptoms. Onset of initial symptoms before age 12 years has been a particularly salient threshold in making such predictions (Loeber, 1988, 1990; Loeber, Green, Lahey, Christ, & Frick, 1992; Patterson, 1982, Patterson et al., 1992; Tolan, 1987). Among the factors that seem to be associated with an early onset form of CD are a prior history of ODD and ADHD in childhood (Loeber, 1990).

## The Prevalence of Defiant Behavior

Undoubtedly, the frequency with which children or adolescents manifest clinically significant and impairing levels of defiant conduct is greatly determined by the definition used for such conduct when surveying populations. The DSM-IV cites a prevalence ranging between 2% and 16% for ODD (APA, 1994). For CD, rates of 6–16% for males and 2–9% for females have been cited (APA, 1994). Using parent reports of child and teen behavior in a large sample (*n* = 1,096) of military dependents ages 6–17 years, one study reported a prevalence of 4.9% for ODD and 1.9% for CD, based on DSM-III-R (APA, 1987) diagnostic criteria (Jensen et al., 1995). When teacher ratings of DSM-III-R symptoms were collected on boys ages 5–14 years, Pelham, Gnagy, Greenslade, and Milich (1992) found a prevalence of 3.2% for ODD and 1.3% for CD. But teachers have a very limited context in which to observe child or teen behavior (school grounds), and opposi-

**TABLE 1.3.** Diagnostic Criteria for Conduct Disorder

A. A repetitive and persistent pattern of behavior in which the basic rights of others or major age-appropriate societal norms or rules are violated, as manifested by the presence of three (or more) of the following criteria in the past 12 months, with at least one criterion present in the past 6 months:

**Aggression to people and animals**
(1) often bullies, threatens, or intimidates others
(2) often initiates physical fights
(3) has used a weapon that can cause serious physical harm to others (e.g., a bat, brick, broken bottle, knife, gun)
(4) has been physically cruel to people
(5) has been physically cruel to animals
(6) has stolen while confronting a victim (e.g., mugging, purse snatching, extortion, armed robbery)
(7) has forced someone into sexual activity

**Destruction of property**
(8) has deliberately engaged in fire setting with the intention of causing serious damage
(9) has deliberately destroyed others' property (other than by fire setting)

**Deceitfulness or theft**
(10) has broken into someone else's house, building, or car
(11) often lies to obtain goods or favors or to avoid obligations (i.e., "cons" others)
(12) has stolen items of nontrivial value without confronting a victim (e.g. shoplifting, but without breaking and entering; forgery)

**Serious violations of rules**
(13) often stays out at night despite parental prohibitions, beginning before age 13 years
(14) has run away from home overnight at least twice while living in parental or surrogate home (or once without returning for a lengthy period)
(15) is often truant from school, beginning before age 13 years

B. The disturbance in behavior causes clinically significant impairment in social, academic, or occupational functioning.

C. If the individual is age 18 years or older, criteria are not met for Antisocial Personality Disorder.

*Specify* type based on age at onset:
  **Childhood-Onset Type:** onset of at least one criterion characteristic of Conduct Disorder prior to age 10 years
  **Adolescent-Onset Type:** absence of any criteria characteristic of Conduct Disorder prior to age 10 years

*Specify* severity:
  **Mild:** few if any conduct problems in excess of those required to make the diagnosis **and** conduct problems cause only minor harm to others
  **Moderate:** number of conduct problems and effect on others intermediate between "mild" and "severe"
  **Severe:** many conduct problems in excess of those required to make the diagnosis **or** conduct problems cause considerable harm to others

*Note.* From American Psychiatric Association (1994, pp. 90–91). Copyright 1994 by the American Psychiatric Association. Reprinted by permission.

tional and antisocial conduct is more likely to occur in the community or at home. As a consequence, prevalence rates for these forms of misconduct based on teacher observations are likely to be underestimates.

For specifically adolescent samples, prevalence rates found in research studies have ranged from 1.7% to 2.5% for ODD and 3.2% to 7.3% for CD, using parents' reports and adolescents' self-reports of symptoms from the DSM-III or DSM-III-R APA (1980, 1987)

**TABLE 1.4.** Diagnostic Criteria for Attention-Deficit/Hyperactivity Disorder

A. Either (1) or (2):

    (1) six (or more) of the following symptoms of **inattention** have persisted for at least 6 months to a degree that is maladaptive and inconsistent with developmental level:

    *Inattention*

        (a) often fails to give close attention to details or makes careless mistakes in schoolwork, work, or other activities
        (b) often has difficulty sustaining attention in tasks or play activities
        (c) often does not seem to listen when spoken to directly
        (d) often does not follow through on instructions and fails to finish schoolwork, chores, or duties in the workplace (not due to oppositional behavior or failure to understand instructions)
        (e) often has difficulty organizing tasks and activities
        (f) often avoids, dislikes, or is reluctant to engage in tasks that require sustained mental effort (such as school work or homework)
        (g) often loses things necessary for tasks or activities (e.g., toys, school assignments, pencils, books, or tools)
        (h) is often easily distracted by extraneous stimuli
        (i) is often forgetful in daily activities

    (2) six (or more) of the following symptoms of **hyperactivity–impulsivity** have persisted for at least 6 months to a degree that is maladaptive and inconsistent with developmental level:

    *Hyperactivity*

        (a) often fidgets with hands or feet or squirms in seat
        (b) often leaves seat in classroom or in other situations in which remaining seated is expected
        (c) often runs about or climbs excessively in situations in which it is inappropriate (in adolescents or adults, may be limited to subjective feelings of restlessness)
        (d) often has difficulty playing or engaging in leisure activities quietly
        (e) is often "on the go" or often acts as if "driven by a motor"
        (f) often talks excessively

    *Impulsivity*

        (g) often blurts out answers before the questions have been completed
        (h) often has difficulty awaiting turn
        (i) often interrupts or intrudes on others (e.g., butts into conversations or games)

B. Some hyperactive–impulsive or inattentive symptoms that caused impairment were present before age 7 years.

C. Some impairment from the symptoms is present in two or more settings (e.g., at school [or work] and at home).

D. There must be clear evidence of clinically significant impairment in social, academic, or occupational functioning.

E. The symptoms do not occur exclusively during the course of a Pervasive Developmental Disorder, Schizophrenia, or other Psychotic Disorder, and are not better accounted for by another mental disorder (e.g., Mood Disorder, Anxiety Disorder, Dissociative Disorder, or a Personality Disorder).

*Code* based on type:

    **314.01 Attention-Deficit/Hyperactivity Disorder, Combined Type:** if both Criteria A1 and A2 are met for the past 6 months.
    **314.00 Attention-Deficit/Hyperactivity Disorder, Predominantly Inattentive Type:** if Criterion A1 is met but Criterion A2 is not met for the past 6 months.
    **314.01 Attention-Deficit/Hyperactivity Disorder, Predominantly Hyperactive–Impulsive Type:** if Criterion A2 is met but Criterion A1 is not met for the past 6 months.

    **Coding note:** For individuals (especially adolescents and adults) who currently have symptoms that no longer meet full criteria, "In Partial Remission" should be specified.

*Note.* From American Psychiatric Association (1994, pp. 83–85). Copyright 1994 by the American Psychiatric Association. Reprinted by permission.

diagnostic criteria (Fergusson, Horwood, & Lynskey, 1993; Lewinsohn, Hops, Roberts, Seeley, & Andrews, 1993; McGee, Feehan, Williams, Partridge, Silva, & Kelly, 1990). Such studies typically find a steep decline in the prevalence of ODD with age but an increase in CD by adolescence.

Sex ratios in research studies have been approximately 2:1 to 3:1 (males to females) for both ODD and CD. Both disorders, therefore, occur more commonly in males than in females, but ratios vary widely as a function of both the age of the teens and the definition of the disorder (APA, 1994; Hinshaw & Anderson, 1996). Some authors have suggested that females may "catch up" with males in their prevalence of conduct disorder by the adolescent years if definitions of CD are broadened to include more female-like forms of antisocial activities (Zoccolillo, 1993).

## The Rationale for Focusing on Teen Defiance and Family Conflict

This program concentrates on those social processes in the family believed to have helped, at least partially, create or sustain the teen's oppositional conduct and its attendant parent–adolescent conflict. The factors that contribute to teen ODD are more thoroughly explained below in the section "The Causes of Defiance/Noncompliance." The teen's resistance to or lack of cooperation with parental directives are among the most obvious products of these social processes. Other correlates and outcomes of these processes of note are maternal depression, parental stress and low self-esteem or low sense of parental competence, parental antisocial personality disorder, marital discord, and even sibling hostility and resentment, to name but a few (Forehand & McMahon, 1981; Patterson, 1982; Patterson et al., 1992).

There are many well-established reasons for choosing teen defiance, and its associated family processes, as the focus of intervention. Each are briefly discussed in turn below:

### High Proportion of Clinic Referrals

First, noncompliance or defiance in various forms appears to be the most frequent complaint of families referring adolescents to mental health centers, especially for boys (Johnson, Wahl, Martin, & Johansson, 1973; Patterson, 1976, 1982; Patterson et al., 1992). Over half of all referrals to such clinics are for oppositional or aggressive behavior, and this figure rises to more than 74% if symptoms of ADHD are included in the analysis (Patterson et al., 1993). While these teenagers may receive various diagnoses of ODD, CD, ADHD, adjustment reactions, and so forth, a major concern of the parents or teachers referring such a teen is his or her inability or unwillingness to comply with directions, commands, rules, or codes of social conduct appropriate to the teen's age group. Parents may complain that the teen fails to listen, refuses to obey, throws temper tantrums, is aggressive or destructive, is verbally insulting and oppositional, is resistant to authority, fails to do homework, does not adequately perform chores, cannot interact appropriately with siblings or peers, lies or steals frequently, or exhibits other forms of inappropriate behavior. However, these behaviors are all violations of commands, directions, or rules that were either previously stated to the child or are directly stated in the particular situation. Hence, noncompliance, broadly defined, encompasses the majority of acting out, externalizing, or conduct-problem forms of behavior seen in clinic-referred youth.

## High Levels of Family Conflict

Second, noncompliance underlies the majority of negative interactions between family members and the teenager. Patterson (1976, 1982; Patterson et al., 1992) and others (see Forehand & McMahon, 1981) have shown that disruptive or aggressive behavior from children and adolescents does not occur continuously nor randomly throughout the day but instead appears in "bursts" or "chunks." These are episodes of high-rate, often intense periods of oppositional or coercive behavior by the child that punctuate an otherwise normal stream of behavior. Research suggests that one of the most common precipitants of child noncompliance or defiance is parental or teacher requests (Forehand & Scarboro, 1975; Green et al., 1979; Patterson, 1982; Snyder & Brown, 1983; Williams & Forehand, 1984).

Such negative encounters between adult and teen may take the form of the interaction shown schematically in Figure 1.2 in many, though not all, instances. The sequence is initiated by the command or request given by a parent typically to have the teen engage in a task that is not considered enjoyable or reinforcing by the teen, such as to have the teen clean his or her room, work in the yard, do homework, perform other housework, or do school homework. On rare occasions, the behavior-disordered teen may obey this first request. This usually occurs when the parental requests involve some very brief amount of effort or work from the teen (i.e., "Please hand me a Kleenex.") or involve an activity generally pleasurable to the adolescent or that may promise immediate reinforcement for compliance (i.e., "Let's go to a movie or video arcade."). In these instances, as shown by the right side of Figure 1.2, the teen probably complies with the request and the family proceeds into other interactions. This kind of compliance may not seem especially important, however, what is significant here is the fact that rarely is such compliance followed by social reinforcement, such as a positive reaction from the parent that acknowledges appreciation for the compliance. When such compliance goes unnoted by parents, it frequently declines in occurrence over time and may eventually only occur when the activity requested of the teen involves something intrinsically highly rewarding and immediately available to the teen. In such cases the adolescent obeys not because of being previously reinforced by the parent for doing so but because the specific activity required of the teen is itself highly reinforcing. Yet only in a minority of instances will a behavior-disordered adolescent comply with the first commands or requests of their parents.

More often the pattern of events is that seen on the left side of Figure 1.2, the anatomy of an argument. Here the teen has failed to comply with the initial request. The parent often

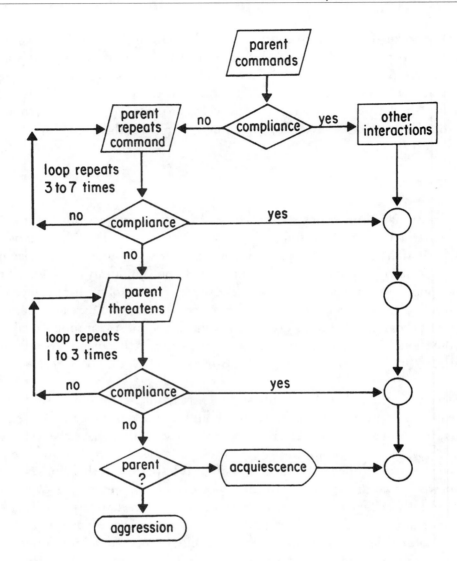

**FIGURE 1.2.** Flow chart showing possible sequencing of interactions between parents and defiant children during a command–compliance encounter. From Barkley (1981, p. 100). Copyright 1981 by The Guilford Press. Reprinted by permission.

simply repeats the request to the teen. This is rarely met with cooperation from the teen and so the request may be repeated again, over and over in various forms yet without the teen complying with any of them. Parental frustration and anger often rises throughout this request–noncompliance interaction, and the emotional intensity of the interaction heightens. The parent may then issue a warning or threat that if compliance does not occur, something unpleasant or punitive will follow. Yet even then the teen often fails to comply, perhaps in part because the parents frequently repeat the threat. The threat lacks credibility and often goes unenforced as well. Not only do the parents' anger and frustration escalate during these encounters, but so does the teen's defensiveness, annoyance, irritability, and anger. Over time, both parent's and teen's level of emotion toward the other escalates, with voices rising in volume and intensity, and further behavioral displays of insults or putdowns, angry refusals, defiance, or destructiveness being made. Ultimately, the interaction sequence ends in one of several ways. Less frequently, the parent disciplines the teen, perhaps sending the teen to his or her room, removing a privilege from the teen, or, rarely, hitting the teen. Such discipline often fails because it is inconsistently applied and delayed well past the point when compliance was initially requested. More often, the parent acquiesces and the command is left uncompleted or only partially completed by the teen. Even if the task is eventually done, however, the adolescent has succeeded in at least delaying its completion, allowing greater time for doing whatever the teen wishes to do.

Parents are often puzzled that the teen spends more time avoiding the requested task, as well as arguing or defying the parents, than it would have taken to complete it. But the parent and teen view the situation from very different points of reference and probably have different perspectives on time itself. Teenagers tend to evaluate events in a moment-by-moment framework rather than as part of a larger picture; they generally do not focus on how it will play out over the course of the day and what later consequences may ensue for their conduct. Adults tend to do the opposite and see the larger picture of a situation. For the teen, then, their moment-by-moment procrastination is doubly reinforcing in this sense, serving to permit continued participation in a desired activity (positive reinforcement) while, for the moment, successfully avoiding the unpleasant task being imposed by the parent (negative reinforcement). The ultimate outcome of the interaction (eventual punishment or forced compliance, diminished parent–adolescent relationship, decreased family recreational time together, etc.) is sufficiently delayed so as to have little, if any, influence on the teen's immediate behavior.

Acquiescence occurs when the teen fails to accomplish the requested activity and the parent simply relents. In some instances, the teen, let's say a boy, leaves the situation. He leaves the room (house, yard) without accomplishing the task. Or the parent storms out of the room in anger or frustration, leaving the teen to return to his previous activities. In some cases, the parent may in fact complete the task him or herself, cleaning up the teen's room, for example, because the parent can no longer tolerate the mess. Another parent may assist the teen with the task after directing the teen to do it. In a few instances, the teen may not only succeed in escaping the task, but may also receive some positive consequence, such as when the teen ignores the request, leaves the house, and goes to hang out with his or her peers at the shopping mall. It is likely that such dual consequences for oppositional behavior rapidly accelerate the adolescent's acquisition and maintenance of such behavior patterns in future similar circumstances (Patterson, 1976, 1982). These acquiescent interaction patterns can be found to underly many of the negative encounters between parents and defiant teens. They must be made the focus of treatment if the troubles of the family are to be successfully ameliorated and the parent–teen relationship improved.

## Situational Pervasiveness

A third rationale for selecting noncompliance and parent–teen conflicts as the targets of intervention is the relatively greater pervasiveness of teen defiance across settings compared to other behavioral problems, such as anxiety. Research suggests that teens who display noncompliance or coercive behavior in one situation are highly likely to employ it eventually elsewhere, with other commands or instructions, and with other adults or peers (Hinshaw & Anderson, 1996; Forehand & McMahon, 1981; Patterson, 1982). Improving teen cooperation and compliance may therefore have widespread effects across many situations and individuals and may prove more effective than selecting one behavioral problem specific to only one situation as the focus of therapy.

## Effects on the Family Social Ecology

The fourth reason to target teen defiance is that the sequencing of parent–teen interactions outlined in Figure 1.2 may have indirect effects on family functioning, and these effects may, in a reciprocal fashion, create further detrimental effects on the psychological adjustment of the defiant teen. The outcomes of impaired family management can be seen in Figure 1.3, as demonstrated in the long-term program of research on aggressive children by Gerald Patterson (1982) and his associates (Patterson et al., 1992). As noted already, out of this impaired family management process, the teen rapidly acquires a set of coercive behaviors to use against the parent and other family members (or even peers) when the teen is instructed to do something he or she does not like to do (Patterson, 1982). Parents may also come to acquire a set of escalating coercive behaviors to use with the adolescent as a result of those rare occasions when yelling, threatening, or punishing the teen eventually led to compliance. Furthermore, over time parents may come to make progressively fewer requests of the teen, knowing in advance they will be met with resistance, argument, oppositional behavior, and conflict by the teen. Parents instead may assume more of the teen's chores and responsibilities or assign them to a more compliant sibling. The latter response may then lead not only to declines in the adolescent's overall level of successful adaptive functioning (i.e., independence, self-care, degree of responsibleness, etc.) but to siblings developing hostility and resentment toward their defiant brother or sister. Siblings, indeed, may come to imitate the defiant and argumentative behavior of their conduct-problem brother or sister because of its apparent short-term success at escaping parental demands. In other cases, parents and siblings come to spend progressively less leisure time and initiate fewer recreational pursuits with the defiant teen, so as to avoid any further unpleasantries with that child. As noted above, siblings may also acquire and frequently utilize repertoires of coercive behavior back toward parents (Patterson, 1982; Snyder & Patterson, 1995; Stormont-Spurgin & Zentall, 1995), especially when parents have employed coercive tactics with all members of the family, not just the clinic-referred defiant teen. Moreover, siblings may learn to utilize aggression and coercion in retaliation against their conduct problem brother or sister, in part out of self-defense and in part because the entire family has trained each other that such tactics periodically succeed.

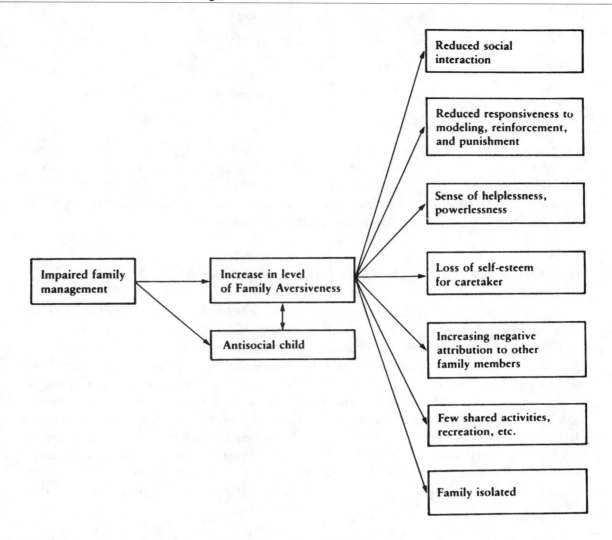

**FIGURE 1.3.** Outcomes for disrupted family management practices and the development of antisocial child behavior. From Patterson (1982, p. 233). Copyright 1982 by Castalia Publishing Co. Reprinted by permission.

Thus, the density of aversive social events within the families of defiant teens is substantially higher than normal. The effects such patterns within a family have on the self-esteem of the parent, on family harmony, on marital harmony (should the teen oppose one parent more than the other), or on the self-esteem of the defiant teen has been substantiated in research (Forehand & McMahon, 1981; Patterson, 1982; Patterson et al., 1992) and almost goes without saying. And so there is a reciprocal system of effects existing within the parent–adolescent relations of defiant teens where the behavior of parent and teenager affect each other bidirectionally while also resulting in broader "spillover" effects into the larger social ecology of the family (Barkley, Anastopoulos, Guevremont, & Fletcher, 1992;

Patterson et al., 1992; Stormont-Spurgin & Zentall, 1995; Vuchinich, Bank, & Patterson, 1992).

## Developmental Persistence

Fifth, noncompliance and defiant behavior in children and teens appears to be highly stable over time, significantly predicting the persistence of this behavior pattern across development (Fischer, Barkley, Fletcher, & Smallish, et al., 1993; Loeber, 1990; Olweus, 1979; Patterson, 1982). Childhood defiance or aggressiveness, in fact, may be one of the most stable of childhood behavioral disorders across development.

## Prediction of Diverse Negative Developmental Outcomes

Focusing the therapeutic intervention on teen defiant behavior is also important because of the repeated association of child and adolescent defiance with diverse forms of later maladjustment during the late adolescent and young adult years (Olweus, 1979; Patterson, 1982; Patterson et al., 1992; Tremblay, Pihl, Vitaro, & Dobkin, 1994). That is, defiant and coercive behavior, especially if it is of such magnitude and duration that it leads to referral for mental health services, is also a precursor or link to the development of other more serious forms of antisocial behavior, criminal activity, and substance abuse (Barkley, Fischer, Edelbrock, & Smallish, 1990; Lahey & Loeber, 1994; Loeber, 1990; Lynskey & Fergusson, 1994; Patterson, 1982; Patterson et al., 1992). The progression from oppositional behavior to violent or criminal behavior can be seen in Table 1.5, where the age of onset of various disruptive behaviors is shown. The pattern here is obvious: there is a de-

**TABLE 1.5.** Median Age of Onset Reported by Parent of Symptoms of Oppositional Defiant and Conduct Disorder as a Function of the Quadrants Displayed in Figure 1.1

| Median age (years) | D: Oppositional | B: Aggression | A: Property | C: Status |
|---|---|---|---|---|
| 4.0 | Stubborn | | | |
| 5.0 | Loses temper | | | |
| 6.0 | Defies, argues, touchy | Spiteful, fights, blames others | | |
| 6.5 | Annoys others | | Hurts animals, lies | |
| 7.0 | Angry | Bullies, cruel | Vandalizes | |
| 7.5 | | Assaults | Steals | |
| 8.0 | | | Sets fires | |
| 8.5 | | | | Truant |
| 9.0 | | | | Swears |
| 10.0 | | | | Runs away |
| Median of quadrant | 6.0 years | 6.75 years | 7.25 years | 9.0 years |

*Note.* Adapted from Frick et al. (1993, p. 330). Copyright 1993 by Pergamon Press. Adapted by permission.

velopmental staging in the relationship of oppositional child behavior to later stages of physical aggression, status offenses, and crimes against property (Frick et al., 1993; Loeber, 1988, 1990; Loeber et al., 1992). Childhood oppositional behavior also significantly predicts later problems with academic performance and peer acceptance (Hinshaw & Anderson, 1996; Loeber, 1990; Patterson, 1982; Patterson et al., 1992; Tremblay et al., 1992; Wells & Forehand, 1985). The risk for later depression, suicidal ideation, and suicide attempts is also greater in children and especially teens with defiant or aggressive behavior (Capaldi, 1992; Patterson, 1982; Patterson et al., 1992; Wenning, Nathan, & King, 1993). Thus, research is beginning to show that the presence of oppositional defiant behavior, or social aggression, in children and adolescents is the most stable of childhood psychopathologies over development and is a more significant predictor of an array of negative social and academic risks than are most other forms of deviant behavior (Farrington, 1995; Hinshaw & Anderson, 1996; Fischer, Barkley, Fletcher, & Smallish, 1993; Loeber, 1988, 1990; Olweus, 1979, 1980; Paternite & Loney, 1980; Patterson, 1982; Patterson et al., 1992). These developmental risks become even more likely and more adverse when child or adolescent defiant behavior is combined with higher levels of ADHD symptoms, particularly childhood impulsivity (Farrington, 1995; Hinshaw, 1987; Hinshaw & Anderson, 1996; Loeber, 1990; Moffitt, 1990; Olson, 1992; Tremblay, Pihl, Vitaro, & Dobkin, 1994). Oppositional behavior is therefore singled out for treatment because of the significant potential it carries for future negative consequences for the child or adolescent if left untreated.

### Prelude to Effective Treatment of Other Problems

Finally, it would be hard to undertake the treatment of any other presenting problems of a conduct-problem teenager without first addressing the teen's uncooperativeness with parents or other authority figures. For example, attempting to tutor a 15-year-old defiant teen so as to help them with their school underachievement is not likely to prove successful until the teen is cooperative with adult requests. This will also be true of noncompliant adolescents who must adhere to other psychiatric or medical regimens (e.g., taking medication for ADHD, management of diabetes, etc.) or educational programs.

## Other Important Aspects of Teen Defiance and Parent–Teen Conflict

A substantial body of research exists on the parent–child and parent–teen relations in families with behavior-problem children or adolescents that is far too great to review here. At the very least, interested readers should pursue the texts by Patterson (1982; Patterson et al., 1992) and the reviews by Hinshaw and Anderson (1996), Lahey and Loeber (1994), Loeber (1988, 1990), and McMahon and Wells (1998). The more consistent and general findings from this research are important to consider in the clinical training of these families. I summarize them briefly below.

Without a doubt, research repeatedly demonstrates that the quality or nature of parent–child or parent–teen interactions is strongly and reliably associated with the severity of noncompliant, defiant, and aggressive behavior patterns in children and teens, the persistence of these behaviors in the teen over development, as well as the risk for later delinquency (Farrington, 1995; Haapasalo & Tremblay, 1994; Lahey & Loeber, 1994; Loeber, 1988, 1990; Patterson, 1982; Patterson et al., 1992; Schachar & Wachsmuth, 1990). Children with oppositional behavior show a poorer quality of attachment relationships to their parents (Speltz, DeKlyen, Greenberg, & Dryden, 1995). The parents of such children also provide highly inconsistent and, at times, even positive consequences to children or teens for their deviant behavior (Dumas & Wahler, 1985; Patterson, 1982). Such poor attachment, unpredictable consequences, and even inadvertent reinforcement of defiant child or teen behavior may serve to increase and sustain occurrences of oppositional behavior in future interactions. When adolescents act out, argue, throw temper tantrums, or directly oppose adult requests, it is surely difficult for parents not to attend to such behavior. Even though negative attention provided by the parents may seem punitive, it may still serve to increase future oppositional behavior in the child or teen (Dumas & Wahler, 1985; Snyder & Brown, 1983). On other occasions, parents may provide positive attention or rewards to defiant teens or children in an effort to get them to stop "making a scene" such as in a store, restaurant, or other public place. Buying a child or teen the object he or she desires and for which has been arguing or throwing a tantrum is but one obvious way in which parents accelerate the acquisition and maintenance of deviant teen behavior.

Conversely, parents may also provide less attention or reinforcement to prosocial or appropriate behaviors of the adolescent. Clinical experience suggests that parents of defiant children and adolescents may monitor or survey their child's behaviors less often than in families of normal children such that they may not always be aware of ongoing appropriate child or teen behaviors (Loeber, 1990; Patterson, 1982). Even if they are aware that the teen is behaving well, the parents may elect not to attend to the teen or praise her for several reasons. One is that many parents report that when they praise or attend to good behavior in their teen it only serves to provoke a burst of negative behavior from the teen. This leads the parent to adopt the attitude of "let sleeping dogs lie" when they encounter ongoing acceptable adolescent behavior. It has not been established that this reaction occurs when parents have tried to praise a behavior-problem child or teen nor, if it does, what the learning history was that established this behavioral pattern. It is possible that parental praise for good behavior in a child or teen prompts the child to misbehave because the child continues to receive parental attention if they do so. Had the child continued to behave well, the parent might have terminated the interaction, moving on to do something else. Another reason parents may fail to react positively when a defiant teen behaves well is that parents dislike interacting with the problematic teen and will choose to avoid interacting with the teen whenever possible. Parents of chronically defiant children or adolescents often develop animosity or "grudges" toward the teen, such that they will elect not to praise him or her when the teen finally behaves well. This may eventually lead to parents' spending significantly less leisure and recreational time with the defiant teen simply because it is not fun to do so.

Parents of oppositional teenagers, especially those teens at risk for later delinquency, may also monitor their teen's activities outside the home less often (Haapasalo & Tremblay, 1994; Patterson, 1982; Patterson et al., 1992) and attend less to unacceptable behavior, possibly so as to avoid further confrontations with the teen. As in the saying "out of sight, out of mind," parents may eventually reduce the amount of effort they spend monitoring a teen's ongoing behavior within the home so as not to have to confront any minor unacceptable behavior that may occur. By overlooking the problem behavior, they do not have to face the aversiveness of another negative, coercive exchange with the argumentative teen about the matter. This may explain the frequent clinical observation that some parents seem to be oblivious to ongoing negative behavior occurring in their presence or are unresponsive when told of such behavior by their teen—behavior other parents would normally react to in a corrective fashion. For whatever reason, some parents of oppositional adolescents are simply not as invested in serving in parental roles to these teens, possibly because of their own frequently younger-than-normal age when becoming parents, their social immaturity, limited intelligence, or even their own psychological or psychiatric disorders. Regardless of its origins, a decline in parental monitoring and management of teen conduct is associated with the development of some of the most serious forms of conduct disorder, which involve both covert antisocial behavior, such as lying, stealing, destruction of community property, and so forth, as well as overt antisocial acts, such as physical aggression toward others (Frick et al., 1993; Hinshaw & Anderson, 1996; Loeber, 1990; Loeber et al., 1993; Patterson, 1982; Patterson et al., 1992, 1993).

Parents may actually also be observed at times to punish prosocial or appropriate behavior by their teen, again because of resentment that may have developed over years of negative interactions with the teen. Parents may often give "back-handed compliments" to a teenager for finally doing something correctly, as when they sarcastically remark, "Its about time you cleaned your room. Why couldn't you do that yesterday?" For all of these reasons, parents are simply not providing appropriate consequences for ongoing teen behavior that would be needed to manage or control it effectively.

This inconsistent and unpredictable punishing of both prosocial and antisocial child or adolescent behavior as well as intermittently and unpredictably rewarding both classes of teen behavior has been referred to as "indiscriminant" parenting, where the teen is damned if they do and damned if they don't comply (Dumas & Wahler, 1985). Dumas and Wahler (1985) have hypothesized that this form of indiscriminate use of consequences by parents creates a great deal of social unpredictability within families and especially in the parent–child relationship. Such unpredictable environments are experienced by both humans and animals as inherently aversive. Any response by the child in such a situation that is instrumental in reducing unpredictability, even if it produces an unfavorable response in the parents, will be negatively reinforced and will thereby increase in frequency. Thus, children may emit defiant and aggressive behavior toward parents because this behavior increases predictability in the course of parent–child interactions. Defiant teens seem likely to have learned the same strategy.

In a somewhat related theory also involving negative reinforcement, Patterson (1976, 1982) has argued that both parents and children in families with behavior-disordered children are negatively reinforced for behaving in aggressive and coercive ways toward each other. Substantial research supports this argument (Patterson, 1982; Patterson et al., 1992, 1993; Snyder & Patterson, 1995). In this theory, the negative behavior of one member of the parent–child dyad serves to terminate the ongoing negative behavior of the other, thereby negatively reinforcing the first member's "coercive" behavior. This type of interaction was documented earlier in Figure 1.2. Patterson has proposed that this may explain why parents and children, once having begun a negative interaction with each other, will escalate their negative behavior very quickly to intense levels of aggression or coercion. Furthermore, the likelihood that such forms of interaction will occur in the future is greatly increased as a result (Snyder & Patterson, 1995).

To appreciate the substantial clinical implications of this theory, it is first necessary to remember that negative reinforcement is *not* the same as punishment—a mistake often made by those less experienced in behavioral terminology. Negative reinforcement is said to occur when, during a situation in which the teen is subjected to aversive, unpleasant, or otherwise negative events, the teen emits a behavior that successfully terminates the ongoing aversive situation or permits him or her to escape from future similar situations. For instance, when the parent attempts to impose the request of doing homework or cleaning a bedroom while the teen is watching his or her favorite TV program or playing a video game, the teen often finds this imposition to be aversive. The teen may oppose, resist, or otherwise escape from the parental demand through arguing, defiance, aggression, or other coercive behavior that delays having to do the request. The teen's success at escaping from the request or directive, even if only temporarily, negatively reinforces their oppositional behavior. The next time the parent asks the teen to do something, the likelihood of the teen resisting the request has increased. The more a parent persists at repeating the request, the more intense the teen's resistance may become, due to this previous success at escaping or avoiding the activity specified in the directive. As already noted, many parents may eventually acquiesce to this type of coercive behavior. Parents need not acquiesce to every command for a teen to acquire argumentative, resistant behavior.

Parents may also acquire aggressive or coercive behavior toward their defiant adolescent by much the same process. In this case, the parent may have been successful, on occasion, at getting a defiant child or teen to cease arguing, whining, refusing, or throwing a tantrum and to comply with a command through the parent's use of yelling, screaming, or even physical aggression against the teen. Parents may also have discovered that rapidly increasing the intensity of their negative behavior toward the teen is more successful at getting the teen to capitulate and obey, especially if the teen initially opposes the command. Hence, in subsequent situations parents may escalate very quickly to intense negative behavior toward a teen because of their history of success at terminating oppositional teen behavior by this means. Parents need not be successful with this strategy during every command–compliance encounter with the defiant teen, or even in the majority of such encounters, in order to maintain this behavior. According to Patterson (1982), only occasional success with coercive behavior is needed to sustain this type of behavior in parents.

Viewed from this perspective, both parent and teen have a prior history of periodic but only partial success at escaping or avoiding each other's escalating aversive or coercive behavior. As a result, each will continue to employ the behavior with the other in most command–compliance interactions. Over time, each learns that when a command–compliance situation arises, the faster each escalates his/her argumentative "in-your-face" behavior, negative emotional intensity, and general coercive interactional skills toward the other, the more likely the other person is to acquiesce to his or her demands. As a result, confrontational interactions between parent and teen may escalate quickly to quite intense, emotional, and even aggressive confrontations, which on some occasions may end with physical fights or abuse of the teen by the parent and counterviolence, destruction of property, or even self-injury (suicide attempts) by the teen.

This view also implies that much defiant teen behavior is not sustained by positive attention or reinforcement from the parent but by negative reinforcement (Patterson, 1982; Snyder & Brown, 1983). Accordingly, when a clinician tells such a parent to ignore a teen's defiant behavior, it may only worsen the problem, as ignoring is likely to be viewed by the teen as acquiescence. In many cases, parents cannot ignore the adolescent because doing so would allow the teen to escape performing the request given by the parent. Parents in such a situation will have to continue interacting with the teen if they wish to get the task accomplished. Many experienced clinicians have noted this problem in training parents of behavior-problem children and adolescents: ignoring defiant behavior is not always successful or possible. Instead, a great deal of negative teen behavior is developed through escape/avoidance learning (negative reinforcement) and is maintained because of its success in avoiding unpleasant activities often invoked by parents. As Patterson (1982) suggests, and as this program teaches, mild and *consistent* punishment (usually time out from reinforcement) must be incorporated into the family training program, as must prevention of the teen from escaping the parental command.

Patterson has also noted (1976, 1982) that parents are likely, once trained, to rely predominantly on the punishment methods taught in the program and to diminish their use of positive reinforcement methods over time. Therapists must anticipate this parental regression and address it during the last few sessions of parent training as well as during follow-up booster sessions. Parents must be instructed that most punishment methods lose their effectiveness when relied upon as the primary management technique with adolescents. Without sufficient positive reinforcement methods being provided for the alternative, appropriate behavior desired from the teen, such desirable behavior is unlikely to be maintained (see Shriver & Allen, 1996, for a discussion of similar problems in classroom management).

This review of several important aspects of parent–adolescent interaction and conflict has a number of implications for the training of parents in effective teen-management procedures, the most important of which are that parents must be trained to (1) increase the value of their attention and its worth in motivating and reinforcing their teen's positive behavior; (2) increase the positive attention and incentives they provide for compliance while decreasing the inadvertent punishment they provide for occasional compliance; (3) decrease the amount of inadvertent positive attention they provide to negative teen behavior; (4) increase the use of immediate and consistent mild punishment for occurrences of teen noncompliance; (5) insure that escape from the activity being imposed upon the teen occurs as little as possible (i.e., the request is eventually complied with by the teen); (6) reduce the frequency of repeat commands parents employ so as to avoid delays to consequences (act don't yak); (7) recognize and rapidly terminate escalating and confronting negative interactions with the teen; (8) insure that the parents do not regress to a predominantly punitive management strategy once training has been completed; (9) train both parents and the teen in more effective problem-solving and conflict negotiation skills; (10) attempt to reform both parent and teen negative communication styles; and (11) when necessary, identify, reframe, or otherwise correct unreasonable beliefs about family life and parent–teen relations that are held by both teen and parent. All of this, then, should serve to reduce the unpredictability involved in indiscriminant parenting while insuring that teen coercive behaviors are unsuccessful in their function to escape or avoid parental requests, demands, and commands.

## The Causes of Defiance/Noncompliance

As discussed above, one of the major causes of noncompliance, defiance, and social aggression repeatedly identified in research studies is poor, ineffective, inconsistent, and indiscriminant child- or teen-management methods being employed by parents, often combined with unusually harsh or extreme disciplinary methods and poor monitoring of teen activities (Farrington, 1995; Loeber, 1990; Olweus, 1980; Patterson, 1982; Patterson et al., 1992). As a result, noncompliance and defiance by teenagers becomes a very effective method for escaping or avoiding unpleasant, boring, or effortful tasks, may increase the predictability of consequences in parent–teen exchanges (no matter how negative), and on some occasions may itself be rewarded. But it would be erroneous to conclude from this that all noncompliant or defiant behavior is simply learned out of the parent–teen relationship and its history. While the exact form, nature, or topography of noncompliant and defiant responses and even their severity in a teen probably has much to do with the teen's learning history within a family, the probability of acquiring or emitting oppositional or noncompliant behavior is also affected by at least three other domains of influence (Loeber, 1990; Patterson, 1982). Combined with the *impaired child and family management practices* discussed above (which constitute Factor One). These causal influences make up a *four-factor model* of oppositional behavior in children or adolescents.

## Factor One

The first factor in teen defiant behavior is impaired *child- and family-management practices*, which has already been discussed here.

## Factor Two

It is becoming clear from research that *adolescents having certain temperaments and cognitive characteristics* are more prone to emit coercive–aggressive behavior and acquire noncompliance than are other teens. In particular, adolescents who are easily prone to emotional responses (high emotionality), are often irritable, have poor habit regulation, are highly active, and/or are more inattentive and impulsive (have ADHD) appear more likely to display disruptive behavior disorders and, therefore, to demonstrate defiant and coercive behavior than teens without these negative temperamental characteristics (Loeber, 1988, 1990; Olweus, 1980; Patterson, 1982; Prior, 1992; Tschann, Kaiser, Chesney, Alkon, & Boyce, 1996). While parental psychopathology and poor marital and family functioning may further exacerbate defiance and aggression, negative temperamental features of the child or teen are among the strongest influences in this process (Olweus, 1980) and may be sufficient in themselves to create these risks (Tschann et al., 1996). However, the effects of early childhood temperament may be gender-specific: negative temperament in infant and toddler boys may be predictive of higher risk for later oppositional behavior but in toddler girls may predict a *decrease* in the risk for later aggressive behavior but possibly an increase for internalizing disorders (Keenan & Shaw, 1994; Shaw & Vondra, 1995).

Symptoms of ADHD, such as overactivity, inattention, and impulsivity, are typically considered aspects of temperament when studied in infants and toddlers. Should they persist into later school-age years, such symptoms are more likely to create parent–child and, later, parent–teen interaction conflicts (Barkley, 1985; Barkley, Anastopoulos, et al., 1992; Barkley, Fischer, Edelbrock, & Smallish, 1991; Danforth, Barkley, & Stokes, 1991; Fletcher, Fischer, Barkley, & Smallish, 1996; Johnston, 1996; Mash & Johnston, 1982). Symptoms of ADHD may prevent a child or teen from finishing assigned activities and thus make the teen more likely to elicit increased commands, supervision, and negative reactions from parents. Adolescents with higher levels of ADHD symptoms may also be more likely to respond to these reprimands and parental confrontations with negative emotional reactions. If such reactions allow the teen to escape further demands, according to the above theories of defiance, their use during subsequent commands by parents will be increased and sustained. The co-occurrence of ADHD symptoms, particularly that of poor impulse control, with early oppositional behavior is especially virulent, predicting significantly greater family conflict (Barkley, Anastopoulos, et al., 1992; Fletcher et al., 1996; Johnston, 1996) and worse developmental outcomes (Loeber, 1990), notably in the realm of later antisocial activity, than does either dimension of behavior alone (Hinshaw, 1987; Hinshaw & Anderson, 1996; Loeber, 1990; Moffitt, 1990; Tremblay et al., 1994).

## Factor Three

Noncompliance or defiance in teens may also increase in probability as a result of similar *temperamental and cognitive characteristics in the parents* (Frick et al., 1992; Patterson, 1982). Immature, inexperienced, impulsive, inattentive, depressed, hostile, rejecting, or otherwise negatively temperamental parents are more likely to have defiant and aggressive children or adolescents (Olweus, 1980; Patterson, 1982). This may be because they display inconsistent management strategies, greater irritability and hostility toward their children or teens, and provide less reinforcement for prosocial behavior (Barkley, Anastopoulos, et al., 1992; Mann & MacKenzie, 1996). Through such inconsistent and indiscriminant parenting, then, children experience periodic success at avoiding demands, further reinforcing the child's use of oppositional or coercive behavior and building a foundation for later adolescent defiance and conduct problems. Such increases in child coercive behavior may then further feed back detrimentally to affect parent mood, sense of competence, self-esteem, and even marital functioning in a vicious, reciprocal cycle of bidirectional effects. Parents may also employ coercive behavior with others in the family, providing a model of such behavior for the child or teen to imitate (Patterson, 1982). In particular, the level of maternal depression and maternal and paternal psychopathology, especially antisocial personality disorder or criminality, are significantly associated with risk for childhood and adolescent oppositional and aggressive behavior and later teen delinquency (Farrington, 1995; Frick et al., 1992; Keenan & Shaw, 1994; Olweus, 1980; Schachar & Wachsmuth, 1990). For these reasons (and those noted below for stress events), parent psychological status must be a formal focus of the evaluation of adolescents referred for defiant behavior (as will be discussed in the chapter on assessment).

A further aspect of parental contributions to teen conflict may be a genetically mediated one (Plomin, 1995). That is, parents may possess certain psychological attributes that make them more likely to create a family environment that is prone to conflict. If those attributes have a sizeable genetic basis to them, then there exists a high probability of the children in that family possessing similar attributes. Conflict in such families arises more from the shared genetic similarities than from the shared environment. There is a growing body of evidence that suggests that parent–adolescent conflict and adolescent antisocial behavior more generally have substantial genetic contributions to them that increase with the age of the teenager (Braungart-Reiker et al., 1995; Elkins, McGue, & Iacono, 1997; Pike, McGuire, et al., 1996). Such research suggests that the impact of parental psychopathology on child misconduct and family conflict may not be entirely the result of a direct causal effect of parental attributes on the family environment which then lead to conflict, but may also be mediated by a shared genetic risk for these same forms of psychopathology (Elkins et al., 1997).

## Factor Four

It is also possible that *larger contextual events* surrounding the family, both internal and external to it, create or contribute to increased risks for teen defiant behavior and aggression as well as later delinquency (Mann & MacKenzie, 1996; Patterson, 1982; Tschann et al., 1996; Wahler & Graves, 1983). As noted earlier, maternal social isolation is one such factor (Wahler, 1975), as is maternal marital status. Single mothers are the most likely to have very aggressive children or teens, followed by mothers living with male partners but who are unmarried. Married mothers have the lowest rates of aggressive children, with these associations being moderated somewhat by higher social class (Pearson, Ialongo, Hunter, & Kellam, 1993; Vaden-Kiernan, Ialongo, Pearson, & Kellam, 1995). Marital discord has also been repeatedly linked to child and adolescent disruptive and defiant behavior (Patterson, 1982; Schachar & Wachsmuth, 1990), although debate continues over the mechanisms involved in this relationship. Also noted earlier, family social disadvantage or social adversity is associated with risks for adolescent defiant and aggressive behavior (Farrington, 1995; Haapasalo & Tremblay, 1994; Patterson, 1982; Patterson et al., 1992). These stress or setting events appear to influence teen misbehavior by causing parental irritability and indiscriminacy in teen-management methods. Such parental behavior further predisposes teens to develop or sustain noncompliance or defiance within family interactions.

\*      \*      \*

Figure 1.4 nicely illustrates the relationships among Factors Three and Four and teen defiant behavior. The figure is taken from Patterson's programmatic research on aggressive children and their families (Patterson, 1982). As noted above, circumstances both internal and external to the family may not only contribute to child or teen antisocial behavior but also make indirect contributions through their impact on the child or teen and even family management practices of the parents. Notice also that for some of these circumstances, a reciprocal relationship exists wherein the circumstances may contribute to antisocial behavior in a child or teen and the behavior, once developed, contributes to a worsening of other circumstances, such as marital conflict, divorce, and parent psychiatric disturbances. Although not shown in Figure 1.4, more recent research with ADHD children suggests that disruptive and oppositional behavior may feed back to increase parental alcohol use as well (Pelham & Lang, 1993).

It is all too common for clinicians to observe that many families referred for treatment of a defiant teen have most or all of these predisposing characteristics: temperamental, impulsive, active, or inattentive adolescents being raised by immature, temperamental, or impulsive parents within a family experiencing marital, financial, health, and personal distress, where management of the teen is characterized by inconsistent, harsh, indiscriminant, and coercive parenting often along with reduced parental monitoring of the teen's activities.

## Treatment Justification

Some noncompliant, argumentative, or defiant behavior is normal for children and particularly for adolescents, and should not be thought of as being pathological or abnormal just because it occurs sporadically. Nor will such typical and occasional resistance to or

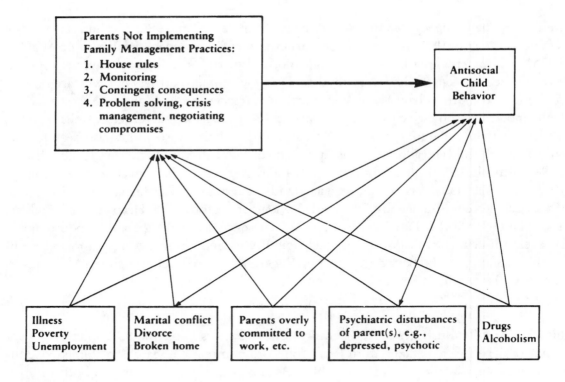

**FIGURE 1.4.** The relations among family management practices, crises, and antisocial child behavior. From Patterson (1982, p. 217). Copyright 1982 by Castalia Publishing Co. Reprinted by permission.

defiance of parents justify a clinical treatment program such as this one. Clinicians must take care to establish *at least two of the following three criteria* for determining that the defiant or uncooperative behavior shown by a teenager is in need of clinical intervention:

1. *The teen's behavior is developmentally inappropriate or statistically deviant* in that it occurs to a significantly greater degree than is common for teens of this age group. This can be established through the use of adolescent behavior rating scales that include "aggression" or "conduct problem" as a dimension of behavior. More will be said about assessment methods in the chapter on assessment. Suffice it to say here that the teen's behavior should be rated at least above the 84th percentile (+1 *SD* above the mean) or higher to establish deviance. Although ratings will typically be created through the use of parent reports of the teen's behavior, given that the home setting is more likely to be where such behavior is at its worst, teacher reports on these rating scales may also be used to establish developmental inappropriateness. Another means of doing so is to find that the adolescent demonstrates, through clinical interview with the parent, sufficient symptoms of ODD or CD as to meet clinical criteria for either of these diagnoses as set forth in DSM-IV (APA, 1994).

2. *The teen's behavior is resulting in an appreciable degree of impairment.* That is, the behavior pattern is interfering with the teen's capacity to meet appropriate developmental expectations for adaptive behavior, such as self-care, appropriate social interaction with family members and peers, acceptance of age-appropriate responsibilities as in chore and homework performance, school adjustment, and the capacity to be trusted to adhere to rules in the absence of immediate caregiver (typically parental) supervision. Such levels of impairment can also be established through some adolescent behavior rating scales that measure dimensions of adaptive behavior or through interviews and inventories that explicitly assess adaptive functioning, such as the Vineland Adaptive Behavior Scale, the Normative Adaptive Behavior Scale, or other such instruments, to be discussed in the chapter on assessment. What the clinician is attempting to demonstrate is that a significant discrepancy exists between this teen's general cognitive ability or intelligence and his or her adaptive functioning as measured by such instruments, which would indicate a social/adaptive disability or impairment in the child. A similar approach has been discussed by others for establishing a social disability in children with ADHD (Greene et al., 1996; Roizen, Blondis, Irwin, & Stein, 1994). For our purposes, establishing that a defiant teen's adaptive functioning places them at or below the 10th percentile for their age would be reasonably sufficient for this purpose.

3. *The teen's behavior is resulting in a significant degree of emotional distress or harm,* either for the teen or, more likely, for the parents, siblings, or peers of this adolescent. Adolescent distress may be established through the use of teen self-report measures of emotional adjustment, such as ratings of anxiety or depression, that convey an impression of the teen's level of unhappiness with the current state of affairs in the family specifically or their social adjustment more generally. Parent distress may be readily established most directly through the use of parent self-report instruments designed to measure this domain, such as the Short Form of the Parenting Stress Index (Abidin, 1986). Distress to peers can be established through rating scales of social skills and peer acceptance completed by parents or teachers.

Regardless of the specific methods used to evaluate these intervention criteria, the clinician must make some effort to demonstrate that the teen's defiant behavior pattern is outside the bounds of normally appropriate teen conduct and that it is impairing the adolescent's adjustment in some way or is creating distress for that teen, caregiver, or others and thus is in need of clinical intervention. Statistical deviance of a teen's behavior alone may not justify either clinical diagnosis or clinical intervention.

Consider the related issue of exactly what should define a behavior pattern as a mental disorder. Out of such consideration may come some guidance concerning the issue of when to treat a teenager, especially one who has not sought out the treatment themselves. As discussed by Wakefield (1992), a clinician should establish that a "harmful dysfunction" exists and is deserving of a label of mental disorder and/or clinical treatment. Wakefield (1992) goes further and requires that an aberration in some internal, normal, mental mechanism must also be present to define a "harmful dysfunction" before a diagnosis of mental disorder is rendered. As Richters and Cichetti (1993) have argued, some defiant or antisocial children may have no evidence of aberrant cognitive mechanisms, although many do (see Hinshaw & Anderson, 1996, for a review), and their deviant behavior may arise as a result of external mechanisms, such as criminogenic environments. These adolescents may not be viewed as having mental disorders. Others disagree with Wakefield's criterion of an aberrant cognitive mechanism (Lilienfeld & Marino, 1995), however, and argue that "fuzzy" boundaries will invariably exist between normality and abnormality. This fuzziness exists by virtue of the often dimensional nature of individual psychological characteristics and behaviors and the arbitrariness of carving nature up to define abnormality along such dimensions (see also Mash & Dozois, 1996, for a discussion of this point).

Although it may be important to define whether or not a mental disorder exists in someone, we are not at all sure that a criterion of an aberrant internal mechanism or even a diagnosis of mental disorder are needed to justify the use of psychosocial treatment for the adolescent and parents, as might occur through a family training program such as this. Some relatively socially benign interventions, such as family training in conflict management, may be justifiable even though some adolescents whose parents undergo such training do not meet diagnostic thresholds for a mental disorder or Wakefield's complete criteria for a "harmful dysfunction." The implementation of treatment, in other words, may not necessarily be dependent upon a diagnosis of a mental disorder, though often it is.

In the end, what this means is that the clinician must stay alert to the occasional possibility that some teenagers and their families do not need specific teen-management training or family training in conflict management. This may result from the fact that some parents, by dint of their own psychological or psychiatric disorders, are significantly distressed by even normal, garden-variety adolescent arguing, misbehavior, or noncompliance. In such cases, it is the parent who may be most in need of intervention for changing their own distress (and developmental expectations of their adolescents) rather than the teen's behavior that is in need of clinical treatment. Milder instances of this phenomenon, where parents manifest no serious psychological disorders, may simply reflect parental overconcern for their teen's adjustment and their own competence as parents. At most, that situation requires simple reassurance by the clinician that all seems well with the teen and that the parent seems to be doing a reasonable job in their role as parent. Likewise, some adolescents may show higher than normal levels of oppositional behavior that do not achieve clinically significant levels of deviance, result in no distress for the parent or teen, or are not associated with significant impairment in teen adaptive functioning. Such adolescents may be viewed as more stubborn, "pig-headed," strong-willed, temperamental, rigid, or opinionated, but those personality descriptors alone would not justify clinical intervention. And there certainly exist those rare cases of adolescents who may be distressed by their own social conduct, even though not clinically deviant in their noncompliance, not viewed as distressing to their parents, and not impaired in their adaptive functioning, as in the case of Social Anxiety Disorders, major depression or dysthymia, or even Obsessive–Compulsive Disorder. Adolescents with these conditions may well be in need of clinical treatment for their own psychological distress, but they may not be specifically in need of a family training program aimed at noncompliant teen behavior as that described here. However, the presence of at least two of the three criteria set forth above is likely to document that a teen's behavior is placing them at significant risk for current and later maladjustment, social and academic failure, antisocial activities, and other significant developmental outcomes that establish the existence of a "harmful" dysfunction even if not associated with an aberrant cognitive mechanism. In our opinion, such adaptational risks justify clinical intervention.

## Summary

This chapter has described the importance of focusing on adolescent noncompliance and defiance as the major target of the family training program to be presented here. The processes whereby teens may develop, maintain, or increase their rate of oppositional, defiant, argumentative, or noncompliant behavior was discussed in some detail, and it appears that such behavior is chiefly sustained by its success at terminating parental demands and allowing the teen to escape or avoid responsibility; such responsibilities are generally unpleasant, effortful, or boring tasks assigned by parents. Escape from those tasks or responsibilities may also permit the teen to continue in a more desirable activity, adding a second form of reinforcement that strengthens teen defiance and parent–teen conflict. Parents may also come to escalate their rates of negative behavior toward the teen by the occasional success such behavior has at terminating ongoing unpleasant teen behavior, such as arguments, tantrums or defiance, and getting eventual teen compliance. Both parents and adolescents may be more predisposed toward such types of coercive behavior by virtue of their particular profile of temperamental patterns and psychological disorders. Larger setting events such as stress, marital discord, parental social isolation, or events impacting the family from outside of it may serve to increase the probability of defiant teen behavior by virtue of the toll these events take on the consistency of parental management of the teen, the positive reinforcement of compliant teen behavior, and the general monitoring of the adolescent's activities by parents.

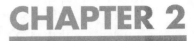

# CHAPTER 2

# Clinical Assessment
# of Defiant Adolescents

Our intent here is not to provide a detailed review of the manner in which a thorough clinical evaluation should be conducted with behavior-problem adolescents and their families. This section, instead, highlights the major topics that should be covered and several methods that we recommend in evaluating oppositional teens, their parents, and the conflicts they experience. We discuss only our recommended approach here. Other methods that may be helpful are covered in the texts by Mash and Terdal (1997), Robin and Foster (1989), Robin (1998), and Barkley (1998), among others.

## Assessment Issues

The evaluation of defiant teens incorporates multiple assessment methods relying upon several informants' observations of the nature of the adolescent's difficulties (and strengths) across multiple situations. Parent and teen interviews are conducted, and parent, teacher, and adolescent (self-report) rating scales of the adolescent's behavioral adjustment are obtained. We also recommend that parent self-report measures of relevant psychiatric conditions and of parent and family functioning be collected. Some clinicians may wish to collect laboratory measures of ADHD symptoms, if that disorder is in question, as well as direct observations of parent–teen interactions. And, of course, teens in whom intellectual or developmental delays or learning disabilities are suspected should receive psychological testing of intelligence and academic achievement if these have not already been performed by the school system or other professionals.

There are several goals to bear in mind in the evaluation of an adolescent for defiant behavior and parent–teen conflict. A major goal of such an assessment is not only the determination of the presence or absence of psychiatric disorders, such as ODD, CD, and/or ADHD, but also the differential diagnosis of defiance or ODD from other psychiatric disorders. This requires extensive clinical knowledge of these other psychiatric disorders; the reader is referred to the texts by Mash and Barkley (1996, 1998) on adolescent psychopathology for reviews of the major childhood disorders and their treatment. In evaluating defiant teens, it may be necessary to draw on measures that are normed for the individual's ethnic background, if such instruments are available, so as to preclude the overdiagnosis of minority adolescents when diagnostic criteria developed from caucasian adolescents is extrapolated to them. At the very least, in interviewing the parent of a teen from a minority group, time should be taken to determine that any symptoms of disorders that are endorsed by the parent are also viewed by the parent as (1) being significantly problematic relative to other same-age adolescents of that ethnic group and (2) resulting in significant impairment in one or more major life activities of the teenager.

A second purpose of the evaluation is to begin delineating the types of interventions that will be needed to address the psychiatric disorders and psychological, academic, and social impairments identified in the course of assessment. As noted later, these may include individual counseling, parent or family training in behavior management, family therapy, classroom behavior modification and curriculum adjustments, psychiatric medications, and formal special educational services, to name just a few. For a more thorough discussion of treatments for childhood disorders, the reader is referred to the recent text on this subject by Mash and Barkley (1998).

Another important purpose of the evaluation is the determination of comorbid conditions and whether or not these may affect prognosis or treatment decision-making. For instance, the presence of high levels of physically assaultive behavior by the adolescent may signal that a parent–teen training program such as this may be contraindicated, at least for the time being, because of its likelihood of temporarily increasing teen violence toward parents when limits on noncompliance with parental rules and commands are established. Or, consider the presence of high levels of anxiety, specifically, and internalizing symptoms, more generally, that may exist in some clinic-referred teens with ODD and ADHD. Research has shown that internalizing symptoms are a predictor of poorer responses to stimulant medication that otherwise is often useful for the management of ADHD (DuPaul et al., 1998). Similarly, the presence of high levels of irritable mood, severely hostile and defiant behavior, and periodic episodes of explosive physical aggression and destructive behavior may be early markers for Bipolar Disorder (manic–depression) in adolescents. Oppositional behavior is almost universal in juvenile-onset Bipolar Disorder (Wozniak & Biederman, 1995). Such a disorder will likely require the use of psychiatric medications, psychotherapy, a family training program such as this one, and even occasional inpatient hospitalization to assist with its management. Finally, more than occasional experimentation with alcohol or drugs by the adolescent would be cause to refer the adolescent to a substance abuse treatment program, after which the family treatment might be resumed.

A further objective of the evaluation is to identify the pattern of the teen's psychological strengths and weaknesses and consider how these may affect treatment planning. This may also include some impression being gained as to the parents' own abilities to carry out the treatment program as well as the family's social and economic circumstances. The treatment resources that may (or may not) be available within the family's community and cultural group should also be ascertained. Some determination will need to be made as to the teen's eligibility for special educational services within their school district if eligible disorders, such as developmental delay, learning disabilities, or ADHD, are present.

As the foregoing discussion illustrates, the evaluation of an adolescent for the presence of defiant behavior is but one of many purposes of the clinical evaluation of ODD teens. A brief discussion now follows of the different methods of assessment that may be used in the evaluation of defiant teenagers.

## Assessment Methods

### Prior to the Evaluation

In our clinics, at the parents' initial contact for an evaluation of their teenager, a form is completed by the receptionist that gathers important demographic information about the adolescent and parents, the reason for the referral, and insurance information that will be cross-checked with the insurance company, when necessary, before the appointment. This form is then reviewed by the billing agent for our clinic and the clinician who will receive this case. Depending upon the clinician's area of specialization, some types of referrals are inappropriate for the clinician's practice and can be screened out at this time for referral to more appropriate services.

At the same time we will send out a packet of questionnaires to parents and teachers to be completed and returned in advance of the scheduled appointment. Parents will not be provided with an appointment date until these packets of information are completed and returned to the clinic. This assures that the packets will be completed reasonably promptly, that the information is available for review by the clinician prior to meeting with the family, and that the evaluation time in the clinic is used in a far more efficient way, particularly given the premium that managed health care plans often place on limiting the time used for the evaluation. Efficiency of the evaluation process is paramount. The packet of information sent to parents includes a form cover letter from the professional asking the parents to complete the packet of information and informing them that the appointment date will be given when the packet is returned. The packet also contains the General Instructions for Completing the Questionnaires, a Child and Family Information Form, and a Developmental and Medical History Form, all of which are provided in Part III of this manual. In addition, the packet includes a reasonably comprehensive adolescent behavior rating scale that covers the major dimensions of adolescent psychopathology, such as the Child Behavior Checklist (CBCL; Achenbach, 1991) or the Behavioral Assessment System for Children (BASC; Reynolds & Kamphaus, 1994). Also sent in this packet is a copy of the Disruptive Behavior Disorders Rating Scale (DBDRS)—Parent Form, provided in Part III of this manual. This scale permits the clinician to obtain information ahead of the appointment concerning the presence of symptoms of ODD, CD, and ADHD in the teen's behavior and their severity; these disorders are quite common among teenagers referred for defiant behavior and so deserve specific evaluation. Parents can be sent a version of the Home Situations Questionnaire (HSQ) developed by Barkley (1990) and modified for use with teens by Adams, McCarthy, and Kelley (1995). The scale can be included in this packet so as to gain a quick appreciation for the pervasiveness and severity of the teen's disruptive behavior across a variety of home and public situations. Such information will be of clinical interest not only for indicating pervasiveness and severity of behavior problems, but also for focusing discussions around these situations during the evaluation and subsequent family training program. This packet should also include both a teen self-report version of the broad-band rating scale noted above (BASC or CBCL) and four copies of the Issues Checklist (found in Part III). The latter scale focuses on a variety of topics over which parents and the teen may have disagreements, assessing their frequency and severity of disagreement. There are three copies, one for the mother to complete, one for the father, and two for the teen to complete (one on each parent).

It is also our custom to send to the teen's math and language arts (English) teachers a packet of forms to complete, with parental written permission obtained beforehand, of course. This packet does not contain the Developmental and Medical History Form. Instead, it contains the teacher version of the CBCL or BASC, the School Situations Questionnaire (SSQ), developed by Barkley (1990) and modified for teens by Adams et al. (1995), and the DBDRS—Teacher Form (found in Part III). When possible, clinicians may find it useful to contact these teachers by telephone for a brief interview prior to meeting with the family. Otherwise, this can be done following the family's appointment.

Once the parent and teacher packets have been returned, the family should be contacted by telephone and given their appointment. It is our custom also to send a letter confirming this appointment date with directions for driving to the clinic. With this letter is a short instruction sheet titled "Preparing for the Evaluation" (also provided in Part III). This gives the parents and teen some information about what to expect the day of the evaluation and may set them at ease if having a mental health evaluation is disconcerting or anxiety-inducing for them.

On the day of the appointment, this leaves the following to be done: (1) parental and adolescent interview; (2) completion of self-report rating scales by the parents about themselves; and (3) any psychological testing that may be indicated by the nature of the referral (e.g., intelligence and achievement testing, etc.).

## Parental Interview

The parental (often maternal) interview is an absolutely indispensable part of the clinical assessment of adolescents. If one were limited to just a single method to evaluate a teen psychologically, the parental interview without question would be the method of choice. Whether wholly accurate or not, parental reports provide the most ecologically valid and important source of information concerning the adolescent's difficulties. It is the parent's complaints that have often led to the referral of the teen, will affect the parent's perceptions of and reactions to the adolescent, and will influence the parents' adherence to the treatment recommendations to be made. Moreover, the reliability and accuracy of the parental interview have much to do with the manner in which it is conducted and the specificity of the questions offered by the examiner. Asking highly specific questions about symptoms of psychopathology that have been empirically demonstrated to have a high degree of association with particular disorders greatly enhances diagnostic reliability. The interview must also, however, focus on the specific complaints about the teen's psychological adjustment and any functional parameters (events that may elicit problem behaviors and their consequences) associated with those problems if psychosocial and educational treatment planning is to be based on the evaluation.

If not obtained in advance, the routine demographic data concerning the teen and family (e.g., ages of teen and family members, parents' names, addresses, employers, occupations, religion(s), and the teen's school, teachers, and physician) should be obtained at the outset of the appointment. This initial introductory period also can be used as a time to review with the family any legal constraints on the confidentiality of information obtained during the interview, such as the clinician's legal duty (as required by state law) to report to state authorities instances of suspected child abuse, threats that the adolescent (or parents) has made to cause physical harm to other specific individuals (the duty to inform), and threats that the adolescent (or parents) has made to harm him or herself (e.g., suicide threats).

The interview then proceeds to the major referral concerns of the parents and, when appropriate, of the professional referring the adolescent. The Clinical Interview—Parent Report Form, designed by Barkley, is provided in Part III and can be helpful in collecting the information discussed below. This form not only contains major sections for the important information discussed here, but also contains the diagnostic criteria used for ODD as well as the other childhood disorders most likely to be seen in conjunction with ODD (i.e., ADHD, CD, Anxiety and Mood Disorders, Bipolar Disorder). This allows clinicians to collect the essential information likely to be of greatest value to them in evaluating defiant adolescents, using a convenient and standardized format across their client populations.

General descriptions of concerns by parents must be followed with specific questions by the examiner to elucidate the details of the problems and any apparent precipitants that can be identified. Such an interview probes not only for the specific nature, frequency, age of onset, and chronicity of the problematic behaviors, but also for the situational and temporal variation in the behaviors and their consequences. If the problems are chronic, which they often are, determining what prompted the referral at this time reveals much about parental perceptions of the teen's problems, current family circumstances related to the problems' severity, and parental motivation for treatment.

Following this, the clinician should review with the parents potential problems that might exist in the developmental domains of motor, language, intellectual, thinking, academic, emotional, and social functioning of the teen. Such information greatly helps in the differential diagnosis of the teen's problems. To arrive at a differential diagnosis the examiner must have an adequate knowledge of the diagnostic features of other childhood disorders, some of which may present as ODD. For instance, many adolescents with Atypical Pervasive Developmental Disorders (Childhood Onset), Asperger's Disorder, or early Bipolar Disorder may be viewed by their parents as ODD or ADHD adolescents given that the parents are more likely to have heard about the latter disorders than the former ones, and will recognize some of the qualities of the latter disorders in their teens. Questioning about inappropriate thinking, affect, social relations, and motor peculiarities may reveal a more seriously and pervasively disturbed teen. If such symptoms seem to be present, the clinician may want to employ the Children's Atypical Development Scale (see Barkley, 1990) at this point to obtain a more thorough review of these symptoms. Inquiry also must be made as to the presence or history of tics or Tourette syndrome in the adolescent or the immediate biological family members. Where noted, these would result in a recommendation either against the use of stimulant drugs in the treatment of a defiant adolescent with comorbid ADHD or, at the very least, cautious use of low doses of such medicine to preclude the exacerbation of the teen's tic disorder (DuPaul et al., 1998).

Information on the school and family histories should also be obtained. The latter includes a discussion of potential psychiatric difficulties in the parents and siblings, marital difficulties, and any family problems centered around chronic medical conditions, employment problems, or other potential stress events within the family. Of course, the examiner will want to obtain some information about prior treatments received by the adolescents and their families for these presenting problems. When the history suggests potentially treatable medical or neurological conditions (allergies, seizures, Tourette syndrome, etc.), a referral to a physician is essential. Without evidence of such problems, however, referral to a physician for examination usually fails to reveal any further information of use in the treatment of the conduct problem adolescents. An exception is when use of psychiatric medications is contemplated, in which case a referral to a physician is clearly indicated.

As part of the general interview of the parent, the examiner will need to cover the symptoms of the major adolescent psychiatric disorders likely to be seen in defiant teens. These are set forth in the Clinical Interview—Parent Report Form provided in Part III. But regardless of whether this particular interview method is employed, a review of the major childhood and adult disorders in the DSM-IV (APA, 1994) in either a semistructured or structured way is imperative to arrive at a reliable and differential diagnosis and the documentation of comorbid disorders. In using the interview in Part III for these purposes, care must be exercised in the evaluation of minority adolescents, so as not to misdiagnose differing cultural standards for adolescent behavior as psychiatric disorders. As we discussed in Chapter 1, the clinician should ensure not only that the behaviors of adolescents are statistically deviant, but that they also are associated with evidence of impairment in adaptive functioning or some other "harmful dysfunction." As noted earlier, one means of partially precluding overidentification of psychopathology in minority children is to make the following adjustment in the Clinical Interview—Parent Report Form provided in Part

III of this manual: When the parent indicates that a symptom is present, follow up with the question "Do you consider this to be a problem for your adolescent compared to other adolescents of the same ethnic or minority group?" Only if the parent answers "Yes" to this second question is the symptom to be considered present for purposes of psychiatric diagnosis. Of course, impairment from these symptoms must also be established before a diagnosis can be made.

When applying the diagnostic criteria for ODD and ADHD (see Chapter 1, Tables 1.2 and 1.4) to defiant adolescents, several problems with the criteria should be borne in mind and adjustments made for them as needed:

1. The cutoff score on the symptom lists was primarily developed on adolescents ages 4–16 years. The extrapolation of these thresholds to age ranges outside of those in the field trial is questionable. Studies of large populations of adolescents (Achenbach & Edelbrock, 1983, 1986) indicate that the behaviors associated with ODD and ADHD tend to decline in frequency over development. Thus, a somewhat lower threshold may be needed for adolescents over 16 years of age if the same developmentally relative level of deviance (93rd percentile) is to be used to define the disorder.

2. The subjects used in the DSM-IV field trial for ODD, CD, and ADHD were predominantly male, by an average ratio of 3:1 (Lahey, Appelgate, Barkley, et al., 1994; Lahey, Appelgate, McBurnett, et al., 1994). Studies of large samples of children and adolescents reliably demonstrate that parents and teachers report lower levels of those behaviors associated with ODD in girls than in boys (Achenbach & Edelbrock, 1983, 1986; Goyette, Conners, & Ulrich, 1978). It is possible, then, that the cutoff point on the DSM-IV symptom lists for these disorders, based as they are mainly on males, are unfairly high for females. In other words, using current DSM-IV thresholds, a girl must meet a higher standard of deviance relative to girls than a boy relative to boys in order to be diagnosed with ODD or ADHD. The critical point is whether a girl demonstrates impairment despite having a lower level of symptoms than a boy. This point has not yet been adequately studied, but a similar argument has been made based on the available research literature on gender differences in the nature of CD (Zoccolillo, 1993). In any case, clinicians should keep this point in mind, as a girl who falls one symptom shy of the diagnostic cutoff score for ODD or ADHD may nonetheless warrant the diagnosis.

3. The criterion that duration of symptoms be at least 6 months was not specifically studied in the field trial and was held over from earlier DSMs, primarily out of tradition. Symptoms of ODD and ADHD are quite common during the preschool years and may persist for periods of 6 months or more without necessarily indicating the presence of a disorder in the child. Also, some research even suggests a large minority (25%) of children initially diagnosed with ODD will no longer qualify for the diagnosis when reevaluated a year later (see Chapter 1). Children

whose symptoms persist for a year or more, however, are likely to remain deviant in their behavior pattern into the elementary school years, suggesting that clinicians might want to adjust the duration criterion to 12 months.

4.  The specific age of onset of 7 years is not particularly critical for identifying ADHD children. The field trial for the DSM-IV found that ADHD children having various ages of onset were essentially similar in the nature and severity of impairment so long as their symptoms had developed prior to ages 10–12 years (Applegate et al., 1997; Barkley & Biederman, 1997). Thus, stipulating an onset of symptoms in childhood is probably sufficient for purposes of clinical diagnosis.

5.  The criterion for ADHD that symptoms must be evident in at least two of three settings (home, school, work) essentially requires that both parent and teacher report sufficient symptoms of ADHD before the adolescent can qualify for the diagnosis. This requirement bumps up against a methodological problem inherent in comparing parent and teacher reports. On average, the relationship of behavior ratings from these two sources tends to be fairly modest, averaging about .30 (Achenbach, McConaughy, & Howell, 1987). If parent and teacher ratings are unlikely to agree across various behavioral domains being rated, this sets limits unnecessarily on the number of children or teens qualifying for the diagnosis of ADHD, due mainly to measurement artifact. Fortunately, some evidence demonstrates that children who meet DSM criteria (in this case, DSM-III-R) by parent reports have a high probability of meeting the criteria by teacher reports (Biederman, Keenan, & Faraone, 1990). Even so, stipulating that parents and teachers *must* agree on the diagnostic criteria before a diagnosis can be rendered is probably unwise and unnecessarily restrictive. For now, clinicians are advised to seek evidence that symptoms of the disorder have existed at some time in the past or present and in several settings, rather than to insist on the current agreement of the parents and teacher.

The foregoing issues should be kept in mind when applying DSM-IV criteria to particular clinical cases. DSM-IV represents guidelines for diagnosis, not rules of law or dogmatic proscriptions. Some clinical judgment is always going to be needed in the application of such guidelines to individual cases in clinical practice. For instance, if an adolescent meets all criteria for ADHD including both parent and teacher agreement on symptoms except that the age of onset for the symptoms and impairment is 9 years, should the diagnosis be withheld? Given the above discussion concerning the lack of specificity for an age of onset of 7 years and ADHD, the wise clinician would grant the diagnosis anyway. Likewise, if a 14-year-old girl meets three of the eight ODD symptoms and all other conditions are met for ODD, the diagnosis should likely be granted given the comments above about gender bias within these criteria. Some flexibility (and common sense) must be incorporated into the clinical application of any DSM-IV criteria.

For years, some clinicians have eschewed diagnosing adolescents entirely, viewing it as a mechanistic and dehumanizing practice that merely results in unnecessary labeling of children. Moreover, they may feel that it gets in the way of appreciating the clinical uniqueness of each case, unnecessarily homogenizing clinical cases. Some clinicians believe that labeling a teen's condition with a diagnosis is unnecessary, as it is far more important to articulate the teen's pattern of behavioral and developmental excesses and deficits than to give a diagnosis. There may have been some justification for these views in the past, particularly prior to the development of more empirically based diagnostic criteria; however, in view of the wealth of research that went into creating the DSM-IV childhood disorders and their criteria, we believe this is no longer the case. This is not to say that clinicians should not proceed to document patterns of behavioral deficits and excesses. That documentation is important for treatment planning. However, there is no excuse for not diagnosing at all. Furthermore, given that legal protections and access to educational and other services may actually hinge on the awarding or withholding of a diagnosis such as ADHD, dispensing with diagnosis altogether could well be considered professional negligence. For these reasons and others, clinicians must review in some systematic way with the parent of each adolescent referred to them the symptom lists and other diagnostic criteria for various childhood mental disorders.

The parental interview may also reveal that one parent, usually the mother, has more difficulty managing the ADHD adolescent than the other. Care should be taken to discuss differences in the parents' approaches to management and any marital problems this may have spawned. Such difficulties in adolescent management can often lead to reduced leisure and recreational time for the parents, increased conflict within the marriage and often within the extended family if relatives live nearby. It is often helpful to inquire to what the parents attribute the causes or origins of their teen's behavioral difficulties, as this may unveil areas of ignorance or misinformation that will require attention during the initial counseling of the family about the teen's disorder(s) and their likely causes. The examiner also should briefly inquire about the nature of parental and family social activities to determine how isolated, or insular, the parents are from the usual social support networks in which many parents are involved. Research by Wahler (1980), discussed here in the Introduction and Chapter 1, has shown that the degree of maternal insularity is significantly associated with failure in subsequent parent training programs. When the mother is highly isolated, it is often wise first to address the isolation rather than to progress directly to adolescent behavior-management training with that family.

The parental interview can then conclude with a discussion of the teen's positive characteristics and attributes as well as potential rewards and reinforcers desired by the adolescent that will prove useful in later family training. Some parents of ADHD adolescents have had such chronic and pervasive management problems that upon initial questioning they may find it hard to report anything positive about their teen. Getting parents to begin thinking of such attributes is actually an initial step toward treatment, as the early phases of family training will teach parents to focus on and attend to desirable adolescent behaviors.

At a later appointment, perhaps even during the initial session of family training, the examiner may wish to pursue more details about the nature of the parent–teen interactions surrounding the following of rules by the teen. Parents should be questioned about the teen's ability to accomplish requests in a satisfactory manner in various settings, to adhere to rules of conduct governing behavior in various situations, and to demonstrate self-control (rule following) appropriate to the teen's age in the absence of adult supervision.

Such an approach yields a wealth of information on the nature of parent–teen interactions across settings, the type of noncompliance shown by the adolescent (e.g., stalling, starting the task but failing to finish it, outright opposition and defiance, etc.), the particular management style employed by parents to deal with noncompliance, and the particular types of coercive behaviors used by the adolescent as part of the noncompliance. This may take 30–40 minutes beyond the parental interview described above, but it is well worth the time invested, especially if parent training in adolescent behavior management is likely to be subsequently recommended for the family. When time constraints are problematic, the HSQ, which was developed to provide similar types of information, can be used. After parents complete the scale, they can be questioned about one or two of the problem situations on the scale. The HSQ is discussed at the end of the section "Adolescent Behavior Rating Scales for Parent and Teacher Reports."

## Adolescent Interview

Some time should always be spent directly interacting with the referred teen. This time can be fruitfully spent inquiring about the teen's views of the reasons for the referral and evaluation, how the teen sees the family functioning, any additional problems the teen has, how well he or she is performing at school, his or her degree of acceptance by peers and classmates, and what changes in the family he or she believes might make life happier at home. A screening for suicidal ideation and substance use should also be conducted. As with the parents, the adolescent can be queried as to potential rewards and reinforcers he or she finds desirable, which will prove useful later in this program.

Children below the age of 9–12 years are not especially reliable in their reports of their own disruptive behavior. This problem is compounded by the frequently diminished self-awareness and impulse control typical of defiant children and even adolescents with ADHD (Hinshaw, 1994). ODD and ADHD adolescents often show little reflection about the examiner's questions and may lie or distort information in a more socially pleasing direction. Some will report they have many friends, have no interaction problems at home with their parents, and are doing well at school, in direct contrast to the extensive parental and teacher complaints of inappropriate behavior by these children. Because of this tendency of ADHD adolescents to underreport the seriousness of their behavior, particularly in the realm of disruptive or externalizing behaviors (Barkley et al., 1991; Fischer et al., 1993), the diagnosis of ODD or ADHD should never be based on the reports of the teen alone. Nevertheless, teens' reports of their internalizing symptoms, such as anxiety and depression, are more reliable, and thus should play some role in the diagnosis of comorbid anxiety or mood disorders in adolescents with ADHD (Hinshaw, 1994). The clinician should inquire about depression, anxiety, and whether the adolescent has any present or past suicidal ideation. It is helpful to repeat the relevant sections of the parental interview for the systematic assessment of mood and anxiety disorders in the adolescent interview. The clinician should also inquire about experimentation and use of alcohol and drugs. Parents may not be aware of patterns of substance use.

Although noting the teen's behavior, compliance, attention span, activity level, and impulse control within the clinic is useful, clinicians must guard against drawing any diagnostic conclusions from cases in which adolescents are not problematic in the clinic or office. *Many* ODD and ADHD adolescents do not misbehave in the clinicians' office, and heavy reliance on such observations would clearly lead to false negatives in the diagnosis (Sleator & Ullmann, 1981). In some instances, the behavior of the adolescents with their parents in the waiting area prior to the appointment may be a better indication of the teen's management problems at home than the teen's behavior toward the clinician, particularly when this involves a one-to-one interaction between adolescent and examiner.

This is not to say that the office behavior of an adolescent is entirely useless. When it is grossly inappropriate or extreme, it may well signal the likelihood of problems in the teen's natural settings, particularly in school. It is the presence of relatively normal conduct by the adolescent that may be an unreliable indicator of the teen's normalcy elsewhere.

## Teacher Interview

At some point before or soon after the initial evaluation session with the family, contact with the teen's teachers may be helpful in further clarifying the nature of the teen's problems, especially those in the school setting. This will most likely be done by telephone unless the clinician works within the teen's school system. Interviews with teachers have all of the same merits of interviews with parents; notably, they provide a second ecologically valid source of indispensable information about the teen's psychological adjustment, in this case in the school setting. Like parent reports, teacher reports are also subject to bias. The integrity of the reporter, be it parent or teacher, must always be weighed in judging the validity of the information itself. Many defiant teens, especially those with comorbid ADHD, have problems with academic performance and classroom behavior, and the details of these difficulties need to be obtained from the teachers.

Teachers should also be sent the rating scales mentioned above. These can be sent as a packet prior to the actual evaluation so that the results are available for discussion with the parents during the interview and with the teacher during the subsequent telephone contact or school visit.

The teacher interview should focus on the specific nature of the teen's problems in the school environment, again following a behavioral format. The settings, nature, frequency, consequating events, and eliciting events for the major behavioral problems also can be explored. Teachers should be questioned about potential learning disabilities in the adolescent, given the greater likelihood of such disorders in this population. When evidence suggests the existence of a learning disability, the evaluation of the adolescent should be expanded to explore the nature and degree of such deficits as viewed by the teacher. Even when learning disabilities do not exist, defiant adolescents with ADHD are more likely to have problems with sloppy handwriting, careless approaches to tasks, poor organization of their work materials, and academic underachievement relative to their tested abilities. Time should be taken with the teachers to explore the possibility of these problems.

## Adolescent Behavior Rating Scales for Parent and Teacher Reports

Adolescent behavior checklists and rating scales have become an essential element in the evaluation and diagnosis of adolescents with behavior problems. The availability of several scales with excellent normative data across a wide age range of children and adolescents, and which have acceptable reliability and validity, makes their incorporation into the assessment protocol quite convenient and extremely useful. Information from such scales is invaluable in determining the statistical deviance of the adolescent's problem behaviors and the degree to which other problems may be present. As a result, it is useful to mail a packet of these scales to parents prior to the initial appointment, asking that they be returned before the day of the evaluation. This permits the examiner to review and score them before interviewing the parents, allows for vague or significant answers to be elucidated in the interview, and serves to focus the subsequent interview on those areas of abnormality that are highlighted by the parents' responses.

Numerous child behavior rating scales exist. The reader is referred to other reviews (Barkley, 1988, 1990) for greater details on the more commonly used scales and for a discussion of the requirements and underlying assumptions of behavior rating scales—assumptions that are all too easily overlooked in the clinical use of these instruments. Despite their limitations, behavior rating scales offer a means of gathering information from informants who may have spent months or years with the adolescent. Apart from interviews, there is no other means of obtaining such a wealth of information for so little investment of time. The fact that such scales provide a means of quantifying the opinions of others, often along qualitative dimensions, and to compare these scores to norms collected on large groups of adolescents are further merits of these instruments. Nevertheless, behavior rating scales are opinions and are thus subject to oversights, prejudices, and limitations on reliability and validity.

Initially, we advise using a "broad-band" rating scale that provides coverage of the major dimensions of adolescent psychopathology known to exist, such as depression, anxiety, withdrawal, aggression, delinquent conduct, inattention, and hyperactive–impulsive behavior. These scales should be completed by parents and teachers. Such scales are the BASC (Reynolds & Kamphaus, 1994) and the CBCL (Achenbach, 1991), both of which have versions for parents and teachers and satisfactory normative information. (The CBCL can be obtained from Thomas Achenbach, PhD, Division of Child and Adolescent Psychiatry, Department of Psychiatry, University of Vermont, 5 South Prospect St., Burlington, VT 05401. The BASC can be obtained from American Guidance Service, 4201 Woodland Rd., Circle Pines, MN 55014.)

The Personality Inventory for Children (Lachar, 1982) may also serve as a broadband rating scale, provided that one of the shortened versions is employed, for convenience; and the more contemporary norms are used for scoring purposes. It is, however, a scale only for parents, precluding the informative comparison that can (and should) be made between parent and teacher reports on the same scale. The recently revised Conners Parent and Teacher Rating Scales (Conners, 1998) can also be used for this initial screening for psychopathology, but they do not provide quite the breadth of coverage across all of these dimensions of psychopathology that the aforementioned scales do.

More narrow-band scales should also be employed in the initial screening of adolescents that focus more specifically on the assessment of symptoms of ODD and ADHD. For this purpose, in Part III we have provided parent and teacher versions of the DBDRS, to obtain ratings of DSM-IV symptoms of ODD, ADHD, and CD. To score the scale items related to ODD (items 19–26), simply count the number of answers circled with a 2 or 3; such answers can be treated as a positively endorsed symptom of the disorder. Items with ratings of 0 or 1 can be considered normal. If four or more items have been circled with answers of 2 or 3, this may indicate the presence of a clinical diagnosis of ODD that should be corroborated through the parental interview form provided in Part III.

For the ADHD symptom ratings, do very much the same thing. First count the number of items circled with a 2 or 3 for the Inattention items (items 1–9). Then count the number of items answered this way for the Hyperactive–Impulsive items (items 10–18). If either list has at least six symptoms answered this way, it may be an indication that one of the ADHD subtypes is present, which should be corroborated through the clinical interview.

Alternatively, clinicians may want to use the summary scores for these sets of items. Norms for such summary scores have recently been collected for these ADHD items by George DuPaul and colleagues (DuPaul et al., 1998). To score these ADHD items on the DBDRS rating scale, the clinician would want to add up *the total points* circled (including 0's and 1's) for the items on the Inattention and Hyperactive–Impulsive lists separately. The 93rd percentile has typically been construed as reflecting clinical significance. Below are listed the thresholds for the 93rd percentile for these scores for each of these lists given separately by source of report, age of the child, and adolescent gender:

| Age (years) | Boys | | Girls | |
| --- | --- | --- | --- | --- |
| | Inattention | Hyperactive–Impulsive | Inattention | Hyperactive–Impulsive |
| | | Parent ratings | | |
| 11–13 | 18 | 16 | 13 | 9 |
| 14–18 | 15 | 11 | 12 | 10 |
| | | Teacher ratings | | |
| 11–13 | 24 | 18 | 19 | 15 |
| 14–18 | 21 | 17 | 15 | 9 |

Another narrow-band scale specific to ADHD is the Child Attention Problems Scale (Barkley, 1990). This scale has the advantage of being drawn directly from the Teacher version of the CBCL and thus benefits from the rigor of standardization and norming that went into that scale's development (Achenbach & Edelbrock, 1986). Its disadvantage is that it does not employ the precise symptom lists for inattention and hyperactivity–impulsivity from the DSM-IV. Thus, high scores on this scale would not automatically indicate a diagnosis of ADHD to be granted just from the results of the scale alone. In fact, readers should be forewarned that scores on rating scales alone are not sufficient to render a psychiatric diagnosis such as ODD or ADHD in a teen. Information from scales must be combined with that obtained from the parent and teacher interviews, as well as the specialized knowledge of the clinician in differential diagnosis, before specific diagnoses in adolescents should be rendered.

The pervasiveness of the teen's behavior problems across a variety of situations within the home and school settings can also be examined. Measures of situational pervasiveness appear to have as much or more stability over time than do the aforementioned scales (Fischer et al., 1993). The HSQ and SSQ (Barkley, 1987, 1990, 1998) provide a means for doing so. Normative information for these scales is available for children ages 4–11 years (Altepeter & Breen, 1992; Barkley, 1990; Barkley & Edelbrock, 1987; Barkley & Murphy, 1998; DuPaul & Barkley, 1992). A somewhat modified form of these scales has been created for use with adolescents, ages 11–17 years, and norms are available (see Adams et al., 1995). The HSQ requires parents to rate their teen's behavior problems across 16 different home and public situations (15 in the case of teens). The SSQ similarly obtains teacher reports of problems in 12 different school situations (14 in the case of teens).

The more specialized, or narrow-band, scales focusing on symptoms of ODD and ADHD (such as in the DBDRS), as well as the HSQ and SSQ, can be used to monitor treatment response when given prior to and at the end of parent training in this program. They can also be used to monitor the behavioral effects of stimulant medication on adolescents with ADHD. In that case, use of the Side Effects Rating Scale is also to be encouraged (see Barkley, 1990; Barkley & Murphy, 1998).

## Self-Report Behavior Rating Scales for Teens

Achenbach and Edelbrock (1987) have developed a rating scale quite similar to the CBCL that is completed by adolescents ages 11–18 years (Youth Self-Report Form). Most items are similar to those on the parent and teacher forms of the CBCL, except that they are worded in the first person. A later revision of this scale (Cross-Informant Version; Achenbach, 1991) now permits direct comparisons of results among the parent, teacher, and youth self-report forms of this popular rating scale. Research suggests that while self-reports of ADHD adolescents and teens are more deviant than the self-reports of youth without ADHD, the self-reports of problems by the ADHD youth, whether by interview or the CBCL Self-Report Form, are often less severe than the reports provided by parents and teachers (Fischer et al., 1993; Loeber, Green, Lahey, & Stouthamer-Loeber, 1991). An adolescent self-report form is also available for the BASC, described above. The DBDRS in Part III can be given to adolescents to complete about themselves (or used as a basis for an interview) as a means of simply gathering the teen's own view of their disruptive behavior disorders. However, norms are not available, so the clinical utility of such self-ratings for the purpose of clinical diagnosis remains uncertain.

The reports of adolescents about internalizing symptoms, such as anxiety and depression, are more reliable and likely to be more valid than the reports of parents and teachers about these symptoms in their adolescents (Achenbach et al., 1987; Hinshaw, Han, Erhardt, & Huber, 1992). For this reason, the self-reports of defiant youth should still be collected, as such reports may have more pertinence to the diagnosis of comorbid disorders in adolescents than does their defiant behavior.

## Peer Relationship Measures

As noted earlier, adolescents with ODD, especially with comorbid ADHD, often demonstrate significant difficulties in their interactions with peers, and such difficulties are associated with an increased likelihood of persistence of their disorder (Biederman et al., 1996). A number of different methods for assessing peer relations have been employed in research with behavior-problem children, such as direct observation and recording of social interactions, peer- and subject-completed sociometric ratings, and parent and teacher rating scales of children's social behavior. Most of these assessment methods have no norms and thus would not be appropriate for use in the clinical evaluation of adolescents with ADHD. Reviews of the methods for obtaining peer sociometric ratings can be found elsewhere (Asher & Coie, 1990). For clinical purposes, rating scales may offer the most convenient and cost-effective means for evaluating this important domain of childhood functioning. The CBCL and BASC rating forms described earlier contain scales that evaluate children's social behavior. As discussed above, norms for adolescents are available for these scales, permitting their use in clinical settings.

## Ratings of Family Conflict

The second half of this family training program will concentrate on teaching parents and their teens problem-solving and communication skills to assist them with negotiating parent–teen conflicts. To achieve that goal, it is necessary first to evaluate the extent to which these conflicts exist, what particular issues or topics seem to trigger such conflicts, and how often and with what degree of negativity or hostility they occur. To do so, Robin has developed a rating scale called the Issues Checklist for Parents and Teenagers (Robin & Foster, 1989). This form is found in Part III of this manual. A description of the Issues Checklist, as well as its scoring instructions and norms are below. Each parent and the teenager complete a version of this scale. Using this scale, the therapist is able to create a hierarchy of parent–teen conflicts that will be used to focus the problem-solving exercises that occur in Steps 10–18 of this program.

In some cases, the therapist may wish to have a more detailed picture of family functioning, including belief systems and family structure variables such as triangulation or coalitions. This picture is particularly helpful in stepfamilies or families with a rigid, authoritarian parent. In these cases, the therapist might administer a lengthy but comprehensive instrument such as the Parent–Adolescent Relationship Questionnaire (Robin, Koepke, & Moye, 1990).

## Issues Checklist for Parents and Teenagers*

This scale was developed by Arthur Robin, PhD, and Sharon Foster, PhD, to assess the intensity of conflicts that adolescents have with their parents. Such information is very helpful in tailoring a family therapy program to the needs of a particular family and in monitoring the effectiveness of therapy. The scoring instructions and norms are contained on pages 61–62.

Deviant scores are considered to be 1.5 to 2 *SD*s above the mean. However, even if the scores are not deviant, parents and teens may still be sufficiently concerned about particular communication problems and conflicts to require some type of intervention.

DESCRIPTION

The Issues Checklist assesses self-reports of specific disputes between parents and teenagers (Prinz, Foster, Kent, & O'Leary, 1979). It consists of a list of 44 issues that can lead to disagreements between parents and adolescents, such as chores, curfew, bedtime, friends, and homework. Parents and adolescents complete identical versions of the Issues Checklist. Adolescents in two-parent families complete it separately for disputes with their mothers and fathers.

For each topic, the respondent indicates whether the issue has been broached during the previous 2 weeks. For each topic reported as having been discussed, the respondent rates the actual intensity of the discussions on a 5-point scale ranging from "calm" to "angry" and estimates how often the topics come up. The Issues Checklist yields three scores for each respondent: (1) the quantity of issues (the total number of issues checked as broached); (2) the anger intensity of issues (an average of the anger-intensity ratings for all of the endorsed issues); and (3) the weighted average of the frequency and anger-intensity level of issues (a score obtained by multiplying each frequency estimate by its associated intensity, summing these cross products, then dividing by the total of all the frequency esti-

*Adapted from Hersen and Bellack (1988). Copyright 1988 by Pergamon Press. Adapted by permission.

mates). The weighted average provides an estimate of the anger *per discussion*, whereas the intensity score reflects the average anger *per issue*, regardless of the frequency with which the issue was discussed.

## PURPOSE

The Issues Checklist is designed to provide scientific information regarding the frequency and content of disputes between parents and adolescents and the perceived anger-intensity level of these disputes. It covers a broad array of possible disputes applicable to 12- to 16-year-old teenagers and their parents.

## DEVELOPMENT

The Issues Checklist was constructed by revising a similar instrument developed by Robin, with issues selected based on literature on parent–adolescent relationships and clinical experience. No pilot testing was done prior to formal validation studies.

## PSYCHOMETRIC CHARACTERISTICS

The reliability, discriminant/criterion-related validity, and treatment sensitivity of the Issues Checklist has been examined in a number of investigations. Estimates of test–retest reliability were computed in two studies. Using small sample data collected over 6- to 8-week intervals from the wait-list groups of two outcome studies (Foster, Prinz, & O'Leary, 1983; Robin, 1981), adolescent reliability ranged from .49 to .87 for the quantity of issues, .37 to .49 for the anger-intensity score, and .15 to .24 for the weighted frequency by anger-intensity score. Parental reliability was higher, averaging .65 and .55 for mother and father quantity of issues, .81 and .66 for mother and father anger-intensity scores, and .90 and .40 for mother and father weighted frequency by anger-intensity scores. Using 33 nonclinic families assessed over 1- to 2-week intervals, Enyart (1984) found somewhat higher reliabilities, particularly for adolescents (range = .49–.80).

Agreement reliability between mothers and adolescents, assessed by examining whether parents and adolescents concurred that an issue either had or had not been discussed, averaged 68% (range = 38–86%). When the congruence of mother and adolescent responses was examined via correlations, results ranged from .10 to .64 (mean $r$ = .28). These results may raise questions about the accuracy of the Issues Checklist as a measure of actual discussions at home or of the recall of one or both people.

The discriminant/criterion-related validity of the Issues Checklist has been studied by contrasting the responses of distressed parents and adolescents (referred for treatment of family relationship problems) with the responses of nondistressed parents and teenagers (no history of treatment and self-reports of satisfactory relationships). Aggregated data from three assessment and two treatment studies with adolescents ages 10–18, male and female, revealed that all the Issues Checklist scores discriminated between groups, with the most pronounced effects on maternal anger-intensity scores (accounting for 48% of the variance in distress/nondistressed status) and paternal quantity of issues scores (36% of the variance) (Robin & Foster, 1984). Adolescent effects were much weaker, explaining 3–19% of the variance (mean = 12%). Across all scores, distressed family members reported significantly more frequent, angrier disputes than nondistressed family members.

When the Issues Checklist was used as a pre–post measure of change, treatment outcome studies of both a problem-solving communication skill training program and a heterogeneous nonbehavioral family therapy revealed significant decrements in anger-intensity and weighted frequency by anger-intensity scores following intervention (Foster et al., 1983; Robin, 1981).

## CLINICAL USE

The clinician can use the Issues Checklist to pinpoint sources of conflict and to survey which topics are perceived as provoking the greatest amounts of anger. These topics ordinarily are selected by family members as their most important problems and often warrant further assessment via interviews and/or home data collection. Ratings of Issues Checklist issues can also help the therapist sequence a skill-oriented treatment so that early intervention sessions focus on less intense conflicts and later sessions address more intense problems. Noting discrepancies between parent and adolescent Issues Checklists and inquiring further about them can also yield invaluable information about differential perceptions within the family system. Preliminary norms from distressed and nondistressed families are also available (Robin & Foster, 1984). Because the Issues Checklist was validated on families with adolescents experiencing externalizing behavior disorders (ADHD, CD, etc.), its psychometric properties with families in which the adolescents have other presenting problems are unknown. Thus, it should be interpreted cautiously with such populations.

## FUTURE DIRECTIONS

The most important unanswered question concerning the Issues Checklist is the extent to which reports of specific disputes correspond to actual disputes. The low reliability suggests that the Issues Checklist may not be an accurate measure of actual interactions. Correlational studies comparing retrospective Issues Checklist scores to daily reports and direct observations of family disputes are needed. In addition, a broader-based normative sample including distressed families with a variety of presenting problems would be desirable.

## SCORING INSTRUCTIONS

This is a measure of the frequency and anger-intensity level of specific disputes between parents and teenagers. Three scores are computed, as indicated below, and the results can be compared to normative data to make inferences about the level of specific disputes for a given family.

1. *Quantity of issue.* Sum the number of issues checked "Yes."
2. *Anger-intensity level of issues.* For issues checked "Yes," sum the intensity ratings and divide by the number of issues checked "Yes" to obtain a mean anger-intensity score.
3. *Weighted frequency by anger-intensity level of issues.*
   a. Multiply each frequency by its associated anger-intensity score.
   b. Sum the products of each intensity times frequency.
   c. Sum the frequencies.
   d. Divide the sum of the products by the sum of the frequencies.

### Norms for the Issues Checklist

|  | Distressed | | | Nondistressed | | | | |
|---|---|---|---|---|---|---|---|---|
|  | $n$ | $\bar{x}$ | SD | $n$ | $\bar{x}$ | SD | $t$ | $r_{pbs}{}^a$ |
| Maternal quantity | 124 | 22.55 | 7.35 | 68 | 17.83 | 7.07 | 3.62** | .25 |
| Maternal anger intensity | 124 | 2.42 | 0.46 | 68 | 1.70 | 0.45 | 11.43** | .64 |
| Maternal anger intensity × frequency | 124 | 2.29 | 2.15 | 68 | 0.83 | 1.08 | 5.21** | .35 |
| Adolescent–mother quantity | 96 | 20.68 | 7.59 | 68 | 18.46 | 7.25 | 1.88* | .15 |
| Adolescent–mother anger intensity | 96 | 2.34 | 0.63 | 68 | 1.77 | 0.49 | 6.20** | .44 |
| Adolescent–mother anger intensity × frequency | 96 | 1.93 | 1.81 | 68 | 0.84 | 0.86 | 4.60** | .40 |
| Paternal quantity | 60 | 18.38 | 5.05 | 38 | 11.64 | 4.63 | 6.61** | .60 |
| Paternal anger intensity | 60 | 2.18 | 0.60 | 38 | 1.82 | 0.57 | 2.93* | .29 |
| Paternal anger intensity × frequency | 60 | 2.39 | 0.64 | 38 | 1.94 | 0.59 | 3.46** | .33 |
| Adolescent–father quantity | 38 | 13.60 | 5.54 | 14 | 10.71 | 4.65 | 1.71* | .24 |
| Adolescent–father anger intensity | 38 | 2.40 | 0.76 | 14 | 1.75 | 0.64 | 2.80* | .37 |
| Adolescent–father anger intensity × frequency | 38 | 2.72 | 0.95 | 14 | 1.88 | 0.69 | 2.97* | .39 |

*Note.* From Robin and Foster (1989). Copyright 1989 by The Guilford Press. Reprinted by permission.
[a]$r_{pbs}$, point–biserial correlation between the particular score and group membership (distressed vs. nondistressed).
\* $p < .05$.
\*\* $p < .001$.

## Parent Self-Report Measures

It has become increasingly apparent that child and adolescent behavioral disorders, their level of severity, and their response to interventions are, in part, a function of factors affecting parents and the family at large. As noted in the Introduction and particularly in Chapter 1, several types of psychiatric disorders are likely to occur more often among family members of an adolescent with defiant behavior or ODD than in matched groups of control teenagers. That these problems might further influence the frequency and severity of behavioral problems in defiant adolescents has been demonstrated in numerous studies over the past 20 years. As discussed in Chapter 1, the extent of social isolation in mothers of behaviorally disturbed children influences the severity of the children's behavioral disorders as well as the outcomes of parent training. Others have also shown separate and interactive contributions of parental psychopathology and marital discord on the decision to refer adolescents for clinical assistance, the degree of conflict in parent–teen interactions, and adolescent antisocial behavior (see Figure 1.3 in Chapter 1). The degree of resistance of parents to parent training is also dependent upon such factors. Assessing the psychological integrity of parents, therefore, is an essential part of the clinical evaluation of defiant teens, the differential diagnosis of their prevailing disorders, and the planning of treatments stemming from such assessments. Thus, the evaluation of adolescents for defiant behavior is often a family assessment rather than one of the adolescent alone. While space does not permit a thorough discussion of the clinical assessment of adults and their disorders, brief mention will be made of some assessment methods that we have found useful in at least providing a preliminary screening for certain parent variables of import to treatment in defiant teens.

These instruments can be completed by parents in your waiting room during the time their adolescent is being interviewed. The forms are not mailed out in advance with the other rating scales because the clinician needs to explain the purpose of these self-report scales to the parents briefly so as not to offend them with the request for such sensitive information. Parents can be told that having a complete understanding of a teen's behavior problems requires learning more about both the adolescents and their parents. This includes gaining more information about the parents' own psychological adjustment and how they view themselves as doing in their role as parents to their children. The rating scales below are then introduced as one means of gaining such information. Few parents refuse to complete these scales after an introduction of this type.

## Parental ADHD and ODD

Family studies of the aggregation of psychiatric disorders among the biological relatives of adolescents with ADHD and ODD has clearly demonstrated an increased prevalence of ADHD and ODD among the parents of these adolescents (Biederman, Faraone, Keenan, & Tsuang, 1991; Faraone et al., 1993). In general, there seems to be at least a 40–50% chance that one of the two parents of the defiant adolescent with ADHD will also have adult ADHD (approximately 15–20% of mothers and 25–30% of fathers). The manner in which ADHD in a parent might influence the behavior of an ADHD adolescent specifically and the family environment more generally has not been studied. Our clinical experience, however, suggests that it can be quite disruptive of family life and parent–teen interactions. Adults with ADHD have been shown to be more likely to have problems with anxiety, depression, personality disorders, alcohol use and abuse, and marital difficulties; to change their employment and residence more often; and to have less education and lower socioeconomic status than adults without ADHD (Barkley & Murphy, 1996; Murphy & Barkley, 1996a; Shekim et al., 1990). Greater diversity and severity of psychopathology among parents is particularly apparent among the subgroup of ADHD adolescents with comorbid ODD or CD (Barkley, Anastopoulos, et al., 1992; Lahey et al., 1988). More severe ADHD seems also to be associated with younger age of parents (Murphy & Barkley, 1996a), suggesting that pregnancy during their own teenage or young adult years is more characteristic of parents of ADHD than non-ADHD children. It is not difficult to see that these factors, as well as the primary symptoms of ADHD, could influence both the manner in which adolescent behavior is managed within the family and the quality of home life for such adolescents more generally. Our impressions suggest that when the parent has ADHD, the probability that the adolescent with ADHD will also have ODD increases markedly. A recent clinical case (Evans et al., 1994) suggests that ADHD in a parent may interfere with the ability of that parent to benefit from a typical behavioral parent training program. Treatment of the parent's ADHD (with medication) resulted in greater success in subsequent retraining of the parent. These preliminary findings are suggestive of the importance of determining the presence of ADHD and even ODD in the parents of adolescents undergoing evaluation for these disorders.

Recently, the DSM-IV symptom list for ADHD and ODD has been put in the form of a behavior rating scale, and some limited regional norms on 720 adults ages 17–84 years have been collected (Murphy & Barkley, 1996a). This rating scale for adults, entitled the Adult Behavior Rating Scale, is provided in Part III. Adults complete the rating scale twice: once for their current behavioral adjustment and a second time for their recall of their childhood behavior between ages 5 and 12 years. Norms for both current scores are provided in Table 2.1, and those for childhood recall scores are shown in Table 2.2. To score the scales, simply total the number of points circled on the scale for each item across the items and check the tables for the threshold representing $+1.5\,SD$ above the mean for adults on each version. The Inattention items are 1–9, the Hyperactive–Impulsive items are 10–18, and the ODD items are 19–26. Again, clinically significant scores on these scales do not, by themselves, grant the diagnosis of ADHD or ODD to a parent but should raise suspicion in the clinician's mind about such a possibility. If necessary, consideration should be given to referral of the parent for further evaluation and possibly treatment of adult ADHD, interpersonal hostility, or even antisocial personality disorder.

The use of such scales in the screening of parents of defiant adolescents would be a useful first step in determining whether the parents have ADHD. If the adolescent meets diagnostic criteria for ADHD and these screening scales for ADHD in the parents prove positive (clinically significant), then referral of the parents for a more thorough evaluation and differential diagnosis might be in order. At the very least, positive findings from the screening would suggest the need to take these high symptom levels into account in treatment planning and parent training.

## Marital Discord

Many instruments exist for evaluating marital discord in parents. The one most often used in research on childhood disorders has been the Locke–Wallace Marital Adjustment Scale (Locke & Wallace, 1959). As noted in Chapter 1, marital discord, parental separation, and parental divorce are more common in parents of defiant adolescents (Patterson, 1982; Patterson et al., 1992). Parents with marital difficulties may have adolescents with more severe defiant and aggressive behavior and such parents may also be less successful in par-

**TABLE 2.1.** Means, Standard Deviations (*SD*), and Deviance Thresholds (+1.5 *SD*) by Age Group for the ADHD Summation Scores for Current Symptoms Collapsed across Gender

| Age (years) | Mean | SD | +1.5 SD cuttoff | n |
|---|---|---|---|---|
| | | Inattention | | |
| 17–29 | 6.3 | 4.7 | 13.4 | 275 |
| 30–49 | 5.5 | 4.4 | 11.4 | 316 |
| 50+ | 4.5 | 3.3 | 9.5 | 90 |
| | | Hyperactive–Impulsive | | |
| 17–29 | 8.5 | 4.7 | 15.6 | 276 |
| 30–49 | 6.7 | 4.3 | 13.2 | 309 |
| 50+ | 5.1 | 3.2 | 9.9 | 93 |
| | | Total ADHD score | | |
| 17–29 | 14.7 | 8.7 | 27.8 | 266 |
| 30–49 | 12.0 | 7.8 | 23.7 | 299 |
| 50+ | 9.5 | 5.8 | 18.2 | 87 |
| | | ODD score | | |
| 17–29 | 6.1 | 4.7 | 13.2 | 271 |
| 30–49 | 4.4 | 3.9 | 10.3 | 308 |
| 50+ | 3.1 | 2.9 | 7.5 | 91 |

*Note.* Data were collected on 720 adults of ages 17–84 years who were volunteers from among adults entering one of two sites of the Department of Motor Vehicles for a new application or for renewal of their driver's license. The sample comprised 60% males and 40% females. The mean age was 35 years (*SD* = 13.2; range = 17–84), mean education was 14.1 years (*SD* = 2.8; range = 7–24), and mean Hollingshead Index of Social Position (for occupation only) was 40.6 (*SD* = 25.8; range = 10–90). The ethnic breakdown by sex was as follows: for males, 86% white, 5% black, 5% Hispanic, 1% Asian, and 3% other; for females, 85% white, 7% black, 2% Hispanic, 2% Asian, and 2% other. From Murphy and Barkley (1996b). Copyright 1997 by Multi-Health Systems, Inc. Reprinted by permission.

ent training programs (see the section in Chapter 1 on "Factor Four"). Screening parents for marital problems, therefore, provides important clinical information to therapists. Clinicians are encouraged to incorporate a screening instrument for marital discord into their assessment battery for parents of adolescents with defiant behavior.

## Parental Depression and General Psychological Distress

Parents of defiant adolescents are frequently more depressed than those of normal adolescents, and this may affect their responsiveness to behavioral parent training programs. A scale often used to provide a quick assessment of parental depression is the Beck Depression Inventory (Beck, Steer, & Garbin, 1988). Greater levels of psychopathology generally and psychiatric disorders specifically have also been found in parents of adolescents with ADHD, most of whom also have ADHD (Barkley, Anastopoulos, et al., 1992; Breen & Barkley, 1988; Lahey et al., 1988). One means of assessing this area of parental difficulties

**TABLE 2.2.** Means, Standard Deviations (*SD*), and Deviance Thresholds (+1.5 *SD*) by Age Group and Gender for the ADHD Summation Scores for Retrospective Recall of Childhood Symptoms

| Ages (years) | Males | | | | Females | | | |
|---|---|---|---|---|---|---|---|---|
| | Mean | *SD* | +1.5 *SD* | *n* | Mean | *SD* | +1.5 *SD* | *n* |
| | | | Inattention | | | | | |
| 17–29 | 11.1 | 6.0 | 20.1 | 175 | 8.2 | 5.9 | 17.1 | 99 |
| 30–49 | 8.9 | 5.6 | 17.3 | 182 | 7.2 | 6.1 | 16.4 | 133 |
| 50+ | 6.1 | 4.0 | 12.1 | 55 | 3.5 | 3.1 | 8.2 | 38 |
| | | | Hyperactive–Impulsive | | | | | |
| 17–29 | 10.7 | 6.0 | 19.7 | 174 | 9.0 | 6.0 | 18.0 | 100 |
| 30–49 | 8.4 | 5.6 | 16.8 | 181 | 6.0 | 5.1 | 13.7 | 135 |
| 50+ | 5.6 | 3.4 | 10.7 | 55 | 3.3 | 2.7 | 7.4 | 39 |
| | | | Total ADHD score | | | | | |
| 17–29 | 21.8 | 11.3 | 38.8 | 173 | 17.3 | 11.4 | 34.4 | 96 |
| 30–49 | 17.3 | 10.4 | 32.9 | 177 | 13.2 | 10.8 | 29.4 | 129 |
| 50+ | 11.6 | 6.2 | 20.9 | 54 | 63 | 4.5 | 13.1 | 37 |
| | | | ODD score | | | | | |
| 17–29 | 9.3 | 6.1 | 18.5 | 171 | 7.2 | 5.9 | 16.1 | 102 |
| 30–49 | 6.9 | 5.5 | 15.2 | 178 | 4.8 | 4.9 | 12.2 | 133 |
| 50+ | 3.9 | 3.6 | 9.3 | 54 | 2.4 | 3.1 | 7.1 | 39 |

is through the use of the Symptom Checklist 90—Revised (Derogatis, 1986). This instrument not only has a scale assessing depression in adults but also scales measuring other dimensions of adult psychopathology and psychological distress. Whether clinicians use this or some other scale, the assessment of parental psychological distress generally and psychiatric disorders particularly makes sense in view of their likely impact on the teen's prognosis and the implementation of the teen's treatments typically delivered via the parents.

## Summary

It should be clear from the foregoing that the assessment of defiant adolescents is a complex and serious endeavor requiring adequate time (approximately 3 hours), knowledge of the relevant research and clinical literature as well as differential diagnosis, skillful clinical judgment, and sufficient resources to obtain multiple types of information from multiple sources (parents, child, teacher), using a variety of assessment methods.

# Treatment Implications

A multimethod assessment protocol for defiant behavior in adolescents will certainly reveal a variety of areas of deficits, excesses, and impairments requiring clinical intervention, and perhaps even more detailed behavioral assessment than has been noted here. The subsequent treatments undoubtedly will be based on those deficit areas found to be the most salient, the most significant to the concerns of the referral agent (e.g., parent, physician, teacher, etc.), or having the greatest impact on present and later adjustment. Treatment recommendations may range from simple parent counseling concerning the disorder, in those cases found to have no impairments, to residential treatment for those ODD or CD adolescents having severe, chronic, or even dangerous forms of conduct problems or depression. Between these extremes, treatment recommendations may focus on improving any comorbid ADHD through stimulant medication or classroom behavioral interventions and improving the oppositional behavior of the defiant adolescent through family training in effective adolescent management procedures and in parent–teen problem-solving and communication skills. Many defiant adolescents have peer relationship problems that might benefit from individual or group social skills training, provided such training is implemented within the school or neighborhood settings in which such skills are needed. The evaluation will, in most cases, reveal the need for multiple interventions for the teen, or even the other family members, to fully address the issues raised therein. Regardless of the treatments indicated from the initial evaluation, ongoing, periodic reassessment using many of the methods noted above will be necessary to document change (or the lack thereof) throughout treatment, maintenance treatment gains over time after treatment termination, and generalization (or the lack of it) of treatment effects to other problematic behaviors and environments.

# Legal and Ethical Issues

Apart from the legal and ethical issues involved in the general practice of providing mental health services to children, several such issues may be somewhat more likely to occur in the evaluation of defiant teens. The first of these involves the issue of custody or guardianship of the adolescent as it pertains to the initial request for evaluation of the adolescent. Adolescents with ODD, ADHD, or CD are more likely than average to come from families in which the parents have separated or divorced or in which significant marital discord may exist between the biological parents. As a result, the clinician must take care at the point of contact between the family and the clinic or professional to determine who has legal custody of the adolescent, and particularly who has the right to request mental health services on behalf of the minor. In cases of joint custody, an increasingly common status in divorce/custody situations, it must also be determined whether the nonresident parent has the right to dispute the referral for the evaluation, to consent to the evaluation, to attend on the day of appointment, and/or to have access to the final report. This right to review or dispute mental health services may also extend to the provision of treatment to the defiant teen. Failing to attend to these issues before the evaluation begins can lead to great contentiousness, frustration, and even legal action among the parties that could have been avoided had greater care been taken to iron out these issues beforehand. While these issues apply to all evaluations of children and adolescents, they may be more likely to arise in families seeking assistance for ADHD and ODD teens.

A second issue that also arises in all evaluations but may be more likely in cases involving ODD or ADHD is the duty of the clinician to report to state agencies any disclosure of suspected physical or sexual abuse or neglect of the adolescent during the evaluation. Clinicians should routinely forewarn parents of this duty to report when it applies in a particular state *before* starting the formal evaluation procedures. In view of the greater stress that defiant or ODD adolescents appear to pose for their parents as well as the greater psychological distress their parents are likely to report, the risk for abuse of defiant adolescents may be higher than average. The greater likelihood of parental ADHD, ODD, or other psychiatric disorders may further contribute toward this risk, resulting in a greater likelihood that evaluations of adolescents with disruptive behavior disorders will involve suspicions of abuse. Understanding such legal duties as they apply in a given state or region and taking care to exercise them properly yet with sensitivity to the larger clinical issues likely to be involved are the responsibilities of any clinician involved in providing mental health services to teenagers.

Increasingly over the past decade, ADHD adolescents have gained access to government protections and entitlements that make it necessary for clinicians to be well informed about legal issues, if they are to advise the parents and school staff involved in each case properly and correctly. For instance, adolescents with ADHD are now entitled to formal special educational services in the United States under the Other Health Impaired Category of the Individuals with Disabilities in Education Act of 1974 (IDEA). This, of course, is provided that their ADHD is sufficiently serious to interfere significantly with school performance. The IDEA entitlement is becoming increasingly understood throughout the United States. Less commonly understood is that such adolescents also have legal protections and entitlements under Section 504 of the Rehabilitation Act of 1973 and the more recent Americans with Disabilities Act of 1990, as it applies to the provision of an appropriate education to disabled adolescents (see DuPaul & Stoner, 1994, and Latham & Latham, 1992, for discussions of these protections and entitlements). Space precludes a more complete explication of the legal protections and entitlements here. The reader is referred to the excellent text by attorneys Latham and Latham (1992) for a fuller account of these matters. Suffice it to say that clinicians working with defiant adolescents who may have ADHD need to familiarize themselves with these various protections and entitlements if they are to be effective advocates for the adolescents they serve.

A final legal issue related to defiant or ODD adolescents pertains to their legal accountability for their actions in view of the argument made elsewhere (Barkley, 1996, 1997) that their comorbid ADHD, which is likely to be present in most defiant children, is a developmental disorder of self-control. Should defiant adolescents with ADHD be held legally responsible for the damage they have caused to property, the injury they have inflicted on others, or the crimes they have committed? In short, is ADHD an excuse to behave irresponsibly without being held accountable for the consequences of one's actions? The answer is unclear and deserving of the attention of sharper legal minds than ours. It has been our opinion, however, that ADHD can provide an explanation for the reasons that certain impulsive acts have been committed but does not cause sufficient disturbance of mental faculties to serve as an excuse from legal accountability, as might occur under the insanity defense, for example. Nor should it be permitted to serve as an extenuating factor in the determination of guilt or the sentencing of an individual involved in criminal activities, particularly those involving violent crime. This opinion is predicated on the fact that the vast majority of adolescents with ADHD, even those with comorbid ODD, do not become involved in violent crime as they grow up. Moreover, studies attempting to predict criminal conduct within samples of ADHD adolescents followed to adulthood either have not been able to find adequate predictors of such outcomes or have found them to be so weak as to account for a very small variance in such outcomes. Those variables that may make a significant contribution to the prediction of criminal or delinquent behavior more often involve measures of parental and family dysfunction as well as social disadvantage, and much less often, if ever, measures of ADHD symptoms. Until this matter receives greater legal scrutiny, it seems wise to view ADHD as one of several explanations for impulsive conduct but not a direct, primary, nor immediate cause of criminal conduct.

In addition to these legal and ethical issues, the clinician needs to clarify who is financially responsible for the adolescent's health care, especially in divorced and remarried families. Often, the mother will bring the adolescent for treatment, but the natural father is responsible for payment. Without such clarification, the clinician may not be appropriately compensated for providing family treatment services.

## Screening Families for Parent Training

No single treatment program is successful for all clients. Recognizing this, researchers have studied those factors that predict success or failure within parent and family training programs such as this. These were discussed in the Introduction as likely predictors of success or failure with this type of family training program. It should be obvious that conditions that affect the parents undergoing training will have some affect on their success in the program. For instance, parental psychiatric problems can interfere with that parent's ability to acquire and utilize the information in the training program, if not attendance at the meetings themselves. Parents who are depressed, actively psychotic, or drug dependent during training will have a difficult time consistently utilizing the procedures with a behavior-problem teen, assuming they can follow them at all. Similarly, chronic health problems that affect parents' behavior may interfere to some degree with effective adolescent management. Although there is little research on this issue, our clinical experience suggests that certain chronic medical conditions such as migraine headaches, epilepsy, and diabetes impair the implementation of the adolescent management procedures. Several parental characteristics that have repeatedly been shown to predict poor outcome in training are depression, marital discord, maternal isolation (insularity) from the social community, and family socioeconomic status (Dumas & Wahler, 1983; Firestone & Witt, 1982; Forehand & McMahon, 1981; Strain et al., 1981). These variables probably relate to outcome in a linear way—the greater their degree or severity within a family, the poorer the prognosis in training. Exercising careful judgment, the clinician must, when these factors are present, decide whether or not they should be addressed (when possible) before beginning training.

In a similar way, certain conditions affecting the adolescent may also impede the successful implementation of adolescent management programs, especially the teen's involvement in the latter half of this family training program—the sessions that concentrate on problem-solving and communication skills. Obviously, the severity of the teen's behavior problems should be considered in the decision to undertake this or similar therapy regimens. When physical aggression and assault are likely, residential treatment may be a more prudent alternative to family training, at least initially. Then, once the teen's coercive behaviors have been brought under control within a more closely supervised environment than the home, parent and teen training can serve as a therapy program for the transition of the adolescent back into the home, as well as preparation of the parents for a successful transition. Adolescents using alcohol or drugs may need intensive substance abuse treatment prior to participation in this family training program. Adolescents with severe language delays or those with significant mental delays may not respond well to this program because of its emphasis on compliance to verbal commands and rules and the ability to negotiate agreements with parents verbally. In our experience, adolescents having a mental or language age of at least 10–12 years can respond successfully to these procedures. Greater time may be needed in working with the parents of such a child, particularly with practice sessions in the clinic, but improvement in adolescent behavior in such cases is certainly possible.

## Feasibility of Homework Assignments and Training Methods

Because the present program contains a variety of homework assignments to be done by parents in the first half of the program, and by both parents and teens in the second half, the clinician must consider how feasible such assignments are for a given family and whether they should be modified to fit the individual characteristics of the parent or teen. Less educated parents may require less reading material but greater modeling and explanation of the procedures to successfully understand them. Parents with sensory handicaps may need special devices for recording their assignments, as in the case of using a tape recorder for recording homework for a parent who may be partially blind or who is illiterate. How the methods are taught may also be slightly modified to fit the unique aspects of one's clinical situation or the family in training. A few parents may even need or wish to record the training sessions in order to review them between sessions. In general, the clinician should be sensitive to the individual and unique characteristics of each family and adjust the homework and training methods accordingly.

## Summary

This chapter has reviewed procedures for the assessment of defiant or ODD teens. An approach is recommended that incorporates a structured interview, the use of rating scales to assess adolescent deviance, parent and teen rating scales of family conflict, and parent self-report measures of their own psychological adjustment. Some of these measures, such as the Issues Checklist, can be taken both prior to and after completion of the parent training program to evaluate improvements in parent–child relations. The assessment also reveals parent and adolescent characteristics that when present may indicate that this family training program is not appropriate, because those characteristics are associated with poor training outcomes. Other parent characteristics have some bearing on how the homework assignments can be individualized to a particular family's circumstances.

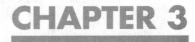

# CHAPTER 3

# An Overview
# of the Family Training Program

In Part II of this manual, we review in detail the specific methods to be taught in each step of the program. First, however, it is necessary to examine the basic concepts upon which this family training program is built as well as the rationale for the sequence of the steps.

## Concepts Underlying Family Training for Oppositional Teens

### Principles of Behavior Management

The first half of the family training program consists of training parents (usually without the teen present) in a series of behavior-management tactics to employ in their interactions with their defiant teen. These principles are drawn largely from the literature on parent training in child behavior management. The principles of child management are interwoven throughout the training program, so practitioners should be sure they understand these principles in advance. They are outlined below.

#### Immediacy of Consequences

Consequences for teen behavior, be they positive or negative, must be provided as quickly as possible if parents are to have any hope of gaining effective control over inappropriate behavior. Therapists need to emphasize repeatedly that parents must provide consequences for their teen immediately after the occurrence of the behavior of interest; they should not wait hours or even minutes to confront the problem or reward the appropriate behavior. Perhaps because of their hectic lifestyles, many parents delay dealing with behaviors, especially positive or appropriate ones. They are often much quicker to attend to undesirable or especially intrusive behaviors. But, even with these, they often wait until after the fourth or fifth repetition of a command before providing some consequence for their teen's noncompliance. In short, the more immediately a parent can provide consequences to a teen, the greater the control they will exert over that teen's behavior.

### Specificity of Consequences

Parents are also instructed that consequences, especially verbal or social ones, should be quite specific. Both praise and criticism should refer to the behavior at issue, instead of vaguely or generally referring to the teenager, his/her general behavior, or his/her personal integrity. Insults and putdowns are not helpful, and indeed lead to greater conflict. Verbal statements to the teen should be quite specific, and any punitive consequences should be tailored to fit the transgression and not be based on the parents' level of impatience or frustration over this or prior episodes of misbehavior.

### Predictability of Consequences

Research reviewed earlier suggests that parents of oppositional children frequently provide unpredictable and indiscriminate consequences to those children. Positive consequences do not necessarily occur following positive behavior and may be as likely to occur following negative behavior. The same applies to negative consequences, which may be provided to the children in an equally indiscriminate fashion. Thus, teen's are damned if they do and damned if they don't. This program will emphasize the need for parents to provide predictable, contingent, and discriminate consequences for teen behavior, so as to decrease parent–teen conflict and make home life far more predictable.

### Consistency of Consequences

Virtually all behavioral approaches to parent training stress the concept of consistency of consequences as a key to greater control of child or teen behavior. This refers to consistency across settings, over time, and between parents. Consistency across settings simply means that if a behavior occurs that is generally punished in one environment, say the home, then it is also punished in other environments, such as stores. While there may be occasional exceptions to this rule, it is generally a good policy for parents to respond to child behaviors similarly across various social contexts. This is often contrary to the practice of parents who handle a problem one way at home and a different way in public places, where others may observe them. Such a practice directly trains the child as to which situation will prove successful for the display of misbehavior.

Consistency over time simply refers to the fact that parental standards about acceptable and unacceptable behavior in children should not vary too greatly from one moment to the next. Although these standards will change as a function of developmental changes in the teen, over more immediate time periods it is necessary for parents to provide consequences as consistently as possible. Teen behavior that is defined as unacceptable on one day should not be arbitrarily tolerated or even reinforced on another. For instance, punishing a teenager for "raiding" the refrigerator because a parent has a headache, while ignoring or actually assisting in such a visit to the refrigerator at a future time, is an ill-advised practice that only greatly reinforces such rule violations in the home. Adolescents readily discern that the parents are not really serious about this rule and that some gambits at breaking the rule may actually be successful. The converse is also true, in that a behavior that is rewarded today should also be rewarded in the future, and should certainly never be punished.

Consistency between parents in the rules they establish for an adolescent and the consequences they employ for the teen's adherence or violation is also important. Quite frequently, mothers tend to manage the problems they experience with a teenager in ways very different from those of the fathers; this often leads to conflicts not only in the development of a consistent set of rules for the adolescent but also in the marital relationship.

### Incentive Programs before Punishment

Punishment for inappropriate behavior should not be introduced in the home unless the parents have established a specific program for rewarding appropriate alternative behavior. Most parents phrase their concerns about teen behavior in the negative, that is, as a form of misbehavior. This naturally leads to a search for punishment methods to suppress the unwanted behavior. As a result, punishment is the main type of interaction between parent and teen; the teen rarely receives recognition, praise, appreciation or other reinforcement for the acceptable behavior he/she shows. Furthermore, we believe that punishment loses its effectiveness in circumstances where the family environment is devoid of positive incentives for appropriate conduct. Having parents propose prosocial or appropriate alternatives to their teen's misbehavior naturally leads them to think of incentives to encourage an increase in the alternatives. Only then should consideration be given to punishment methods for reducing unacceptable behavior. This is especially true in those sessions when punishment is being taught, lest parents think the therapist is advocating the use of punishment as a primary response to misconduct by the teen.

### Anticipating and Planning for Misbehavior

The experienced clinician recognizes that many parents are as impulsive in their reactions to adolescent misbehavior as their teens are in reacting to various events. Thus parents spend a tremendous amount of time managing misbehavior and invest minimal if any time analyzing, anticipating, and possibly preventing problem situations. If parents were to anticipate problematic encounters, they might develop methods that would reduce the probability of those problems developing. Perhaps this apparent lack of forethought is merely the result of being so overwhelmed with incorrigible behavior that it is difficult to "take the offensive," become proactive, and ward off future problems in a particular setting. Or, perhaps, it results from some parents having similar forms of psychopathology to those of their children (i.e., ADHD and ODD) making the parent more impulsive and immature compared to other parents, in much the same way that the teen is relative to his/her peers. In either case, a lack of forethought contributes to many of the difficulties parents have in dealing with children, especially outside the home such as in stores, restaurants, and the like. It is necessary periodically to discuss with parents the issue of thinking ahead and preparing a plan of behavior management for the teen before the family enters a potential problem situation. In dealing with defiant teens, if the parents simply wait until the disruptive or unmanageable behavior occurs and try to determine what to do about it then, it will be too little, too late.

### Reciprocity of Family Interactions

Another concept conveyed to parents throughout the program is that of the reciprocity of interactions within families. Parents often have a unilateral view of the causes of teen behavior problems: it is either entirely the parents' or entirely the child's fault. The clinician must periodically emphasize that interaction patterns within families are quite complex and are not especially well understood at this time. What is known strongly indicates that parents' behavior toward a child is partly a function of the following: the child's behavior toward them; the child's temperament, physical characteristics, and abilities; and prior experiences with that child (Bell & Harper, 1977; Patterson, 1982). Similarly, the teen's behavior is partly a function of how the parent treats the teen; the parent's own temperament, physical characteristics, and abilities; and prior experiences with that parent. Because of this bidirectional influence between parent and teen, it is difficult to assign blame to either party for the current state of conflict. Hence, no time in this program is spent blaming parents *or* adolescents for interaction problems—a practice that has no constructive value in overcoming those problems. Instead, all parties to the problematic interaction bear some responsibility for its resolution. That parents are initially chosen as the major focus of change has more to do with convenience, their greater motivation, and their greater likelihood of cooperation or readiness for change in altering the problem interactions than it does with finding fault with their management skills.

In summary, several general concepts concerning teen management deserve periodic emphasis throughout the course of therapy: (1) immediacy and specificity of consequences; (2) consistency of consequences across settings, over time, and between parents; (3) predictability and discriminacy of consequences; (4) establishing incentive programs for appropriate behavior before implementing punishment methods for unacceptable behavior; (5) anticipating potential problem situations and preparing a plan of action ahead of time; and (6) emphasizing that interaction patterns in families are reciprocal systems, making finding fault with parents or adolescents of little constructive value.

## Principles Behind Problem-Solving Communication Training (PSCT)

The second half of this family training program focuses on teaching both the parents and the adolescent methods of proper problem solving and skills in communicating with each other during negotiations over conflicts. Several principles underlie this approach to family training that should be appreciated before undertaking this part of the program.

### Gradually Grant Increasing Independence

Becoming independent from the family is the primary developmental task of adolescence. Children go from being highly dependent on their parents prior to adolescence to being relatively independent of their parents by young adulthood. Even in the absence of the entrenched defiant behavior of the type dealt with in this program, there is a certain amount of conflict that is normal, as young adolescents individuate from their parents. To prepare adolescents in assuming increased independence responsibly, it is best for parents to grant it gradually. With each bit of increased independence from parental restrictions comes the responsibility to handle this independence appropriately. Thus, parents need to think in terms of giving increased freedom in return for increased demonstrations of responsibility. In essence, they are moving away from a strictly autocratic approach to parenting and toward a more democratic approach. Parents need to plan this gradual granting of increased independence consciously, and to be prepared to pull back a little bit (but not all of the way) when adolescents inevitably make mistakes in handling their newfound freedoms.

Gradually granting more freedom can best be thought of as a behavioral shaping process. A parent might break the terminal independence response into small units, shape each behavior, and then move on to the next step once the teenager has demonstrated responsibility on the previous step. For example, one terminal behavior might be staying alone in the house for a weekend and taking proper care of the house, for example, nothing is left unlocked, nothing is missing, the lawn is watered and pets fed, no wild parties, and so forth. The parent might break this terminal behavior down into smaller units, such as staying in the house for an evening, a whole night, two nights, and so on. As the adolescent successfully accomplishes each step, the parent moves on to the next step. If the adolescent fails to accomplish one step successfully, the parent goes back to the previous step, and at a later time again attempts to advance to the next step in the shaping program. The steps of problem solving, which comprise a major portion of the second half of this intervention program, represent one method for the therapist to teach parents to give their adolescents increased independence gradually in return for demonstrations of responsibility.

## Distinguish Negotiable from Nonnegotiable Issues

Regarding discipline, parents need to divide the world of issues into those which can be negotiated and those which cannot. This is a very important distinction. Parents do not negotiate with their adolescent about using alcohol, drugs, or smoking, or about treating parents respectfully and refraining from physical violence; they set and enforce limits. Each family has a small set of bottom-line issues that relate to basic rules for living in civilized society, values, morality, and legality, which are not subject to negotiation. Such issues usually include drugs, alcohol, aspects of sexuality, religion, respect, violence, and perhaps others. Each parent needs to list his/her basic house rules clearly and present to the teenager those issues that are nonnegotiable. Then they need to enforce the rules around these issues consistently and fairly, using all of the behavior-management techniques discussed in the first half of this program. These issues are not appropriate topics for problem solving, although the principles of positive communication taught in the second half of this program are relevant to holding family discussions on nonnegotiable topics.

The remaining issues not on the list of house rules are legitimate topics for negotiating compromise solutions using the steps of problem solving.

### Involve Adolescents in Problem Solving for Negotiable Issues

Parents need to involve their teenagers in decision making regarding the issues that can be negotiated. This is the single most important principle of parenting an adolescent and is one of the primary methods of shaping responsible independence. Teenagers are more likely to comply with rules and regulations that they helped to create. Furthermore, they may have a novel and creative perspective on the issue because of their youth and unique position in the family. Often their perspective leads them to suggest novel solutions. Problem-solving training is the primary technique for involving adolescents in decision making. Parents need to remember, however, that the teen's involvement in decision making doesn't necessarily mean always being an equal partner with parents, and certainly does not mean dictating to parents. In some cases, parents may retain the ultimate veto over decisions. In other cases, adolescents may be equal partners with parents. Parents need to increase the degree of involvement they give teenagers in decision making gradually, through a shaping process. In those cases where defiant teenagers are already attempting to coerce their parents to do things for them or are dictating to parents, principles of behavior management may need to be used to reestablish an appropriate degree of parental authority before teenagers can be meaningfully involved in decision making.

### Maintain Good Communication

Communication is the glue that binds relationships together. It is very easy for defiant teens and their parents to become embroiled in endless cycles of accusatory–defensive communication, to the point where they are side-tracked from the issues at hand. Defiant adolescents tell their parents very little about what they are thinking and feeling, and parents tend not to listen when adolescents need to talk. It is very difficult for families to use problem solving to negotiate disagreements when the way they talk to each other gets them so angry that they forget what it is they are talking about. Maintaining good communication and, more commonly, replacing negative with positive communication habits is a basic goal of the second part of this program. The therapist will help the family analyze the specific negative communication habits and will employ instructions, modeling, behavior rehearsal, and feedback to teach family members how and when to use positive communication. The therapist will also help the parents to learn to listen to their teenager, and the teenager to learn to express his/her positive and negative feelings and ideas to the parents respectfully but assertively.

### Develop Realistic Expectations

After living with defiant teens for a number of years, it is easy for parents to begin to "think the worst" and attribute their adolescent's behavior to malicious motives. Because these teens disobey so many rules and argue so incessantly, many parents come to believe that if they give their teenagers more freedom, the teenager will inevitably make serious mistakes and ruin his or her life. In the extreme, we call such parents' thinking "ruination." Although this occasionally may be true, typically it is an exaggeration that can become a self-fulfilling prophecy, in that adolescents who know their parents will always think the worst of them may misbehave because they figure "they are damned if they do and damned if they don't."

In addition, when the adolescent inevitably makes poor decisions or acts coercively, some parents consistently attribute these actions to malicious intent, that is, their adolescent is misbehaving on purpose to annoy or anger the parent. Other parents have lifelong expectations that their children should always obey them, and when their children enter adolescence and become more disobedient, such parents respond in a highly punitive manner, spurring rapid escalation of defiant behavior.

We find that extreme thinking along the themes of ruination, malicious intent, and disobedience adds fuel to the fire of defiance and considerably worsens family conflict. Individuals who adhere rigidly to absolutist and possibly distorted beliefs will have a difficult time consistently and dispassionately applying behavior management and problem-solving techniques. In fact, they may resist implementing these techniques. Thus, one important goal of the second portion of this treatment program is to identify extreme thinking and help modify it.

Adolescents also may adhere to extreme beliefs, which need to be addressed as well. Most commonly, adolescents adhere to the "unfairness triad" of beliefs: ruination, unfairness, and autonomy. Unfairness refers to the belief that parental rules are intrinsically unfair and arbitrary; ruination refers to the belief that parental rules will ruin all of the teenager's fun; and autonomy refers to the belief that the adolescent should have total and complete freedom from parental restrictions. Teenagers who adhere rigidly to these beliefs experience more conflict with their parents than teens whose expectations are more flexible (Robin et al., 1990).

### Respect Family Structure

All families have "pecking orders," or hierarchies, and in most families parents are supposed to be in charge of children or higher in the hierarchy than children. In many family patterns, coalitions and triangulation develop. A coalition refers to two people taking sides against a third, while triangulation refers to two people putting the third in the middle, and the third vacillating between siding with one or the other individual. The clinician wants to encourage parents to be in a coalition against the adolescent—that is, to work consistently as a team—but cross-generational coalitions between the adolescent and one parent against the other parent may pose problems. Triangulation may also pose problems, as when an adolescent and a stepparent put a natural parent in the middle, forcing side taking.

The astute clinician needs to understand and respect the hierarchy within a family in order to intervene effectively with family treatments such as problem solving, communication training, and cognitive restructuring. For example, in a stepfamily the adolescent and the natural parent may be in a coalition against the stepparent. If the clinician fails to take this into account and assigns homework for the stepparent to do with the adolescent, the family may not comply with the assignment. Sometimes a single mother will bring in an adolescent, but the two of them live with the grandmother, and it turns out that the grandmother is in charge of the family. If the clinician fails to include the grandmother appropriately in the family treatment, problems may arise.

## The Sequence of Steps within the Program

There are 18 steps to the family training program. The program can be taught as one self-contained unit, with therapy terminating after the final session, or it can be integrated into an ongoing family therapy or parent counseling program designed to address other difficulties in the family, marriage, or parents' own personal life. In some cases, it may be necessary to begin other forms of therapy after these steps are completed, to address other problems of the teen such as noncompliance with medical treatments or poor school performance. In any case, the sequence of the procedures within this core program should remain essentially the same. Much research and clinical experience has been invested in constructing the steps of the program and their sequence, and they are deliberately presented in this order for important reasons.

The initial sessions emphasize ways that parents can deal with their teen so as to regain some control or influence over teen behavior. This is basic contingency management, designed to help parents reassert their authority in the family. It needs to be in place before proceeding to teach parents and teens ways of negotiating conflicts. The development of positive behavior management methods within the family, especially the use of incentives for compliance with rules and commands, comes first; later sessions deal specifically with punishment techniques. Then, in the second half of the training program, therapy focuses on interpersonal skills needed by the parents and teen to develop better conflict resolution. Inverting the sequence such that PSCT is taught first may result in parents trying to negotiate with a teen issues over which they have no immediate control or authority. By having the parents establish their control over household consequences for the teen, at least to the extent that they do control them, parents can provide a home environment rich with incentives for appropriate behavior, but also one in which selective, mild punishment occurs for misconduct. All of this is predicated on our belief that teens are not equal partners in the management of the household or family, nor are they fully cognitively mature enough to exercise complete decision making over their own activities. Parents continue to have some authority and influence in enforcing household rules and expectations for the teen's responsible conduct for as long as the teen is in residence with the family.

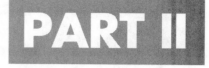

# Session Instructions

*This section provides detailed guidelines for conducting each step of the parent training program. Within each step, goals of that step are specifically stated, an outline for use in the session is provided, and specific instructions for conducting that step are then described. You will want to review the sequence of activities for each session, as described in Chapter 3 of Part I, before beginning treatment with each new case. You will also find it helpful to refer to the outline provided for each step while conducting that step of the program, so as to ensure that all of the important information is reviewed with the parents. Finally, the parent handouts that accompany each step are set forth in Part IV of this manual. These can be photocopied as needed for distribution to your clients as part of your treatment of them with this program.*

# Discussion of ADHD and ODD

## Goals

1. To make sure that parents have realistic expectations for the program.
2. To increase parental knowledge about ADHD if their teen has this diagnosis.
3. To increase parental knowledge of the disruptive behavior disorders such as ODD and CD.

## Materials Required

- Videotapes on ADHD and ODD (to be returned by next session)

## Session Outline

- Review general procedures.
- Outline the major aspects of the program.
- Provide an overview of ADHD.
- Provide an overview of the disruptive behavior disorders such as ODD and CD.

## Homework

- Watch the ADHD and ODD videos.

## Review of General Procedures

Inform parents that you will be meeting for a total of 18 sessions: nine with the parents alone, preferably on a weekly basis, and nine with the parents and teenager together. Discuss fees, scheduling, emergency telephone arrangements, confidentiality and its exceptions, and any other office procedures specific to your practice.

## The Major Aspects of the Program

Briefly summarize for parents what will be covered in each session. Sessions 1 and 2 lay the conceptual foundation upon which specific behavior-management techniques are built, including an overview of ADHD and the disruptive behavior disorders, a model of teen misbehavior, and behavior management principles. Sessions 3, 4, and 5 emphasize the use of incentives and reward strategies for appropriate behavior. Sessions 6 and 7 cover the use of discipline in the form of privilege removal and grounding. Session 8 integrates the program thus far into a set of behavioral contracts or a point system. Session 9 covers school-related concerns. Session 10 introduces the second half of the program, which focuses on problem-solving skills, communication skills, and unreasonable beliefs that may fuel family conflict. Family members are also given an opportunity to ask questions about ADHD if it is relevant for them. Sessions 11 and 12 cover problem-solving techniques. Sessions 13 and 14 continue with problem solving and also cover improving communication habits. Session 15 introduces the topic of unreasonable beliefs. Sessions 16, 17, and 18 integrate all of the above.

You should emphasize to families that success requires not only regular attendance, but also intensive home practice of techniques. Therefore, they will have homework for every session, including the use of a tape recorder during the second half of the program to record problem-solving discussions at home. Families need to understand that although there is nothing magical about this treatment, they will gain far more from it if they practice what they learn.

## Overview of ADHD

If the teen has been diagnosed with ADHD, then briefly review the history of the disorder (see Barkley, 1998). Discuss the three primary symptoms (hyperactivity, impulsivity, and inattentiveness), emphasizing the developmental nature of ADHD and its typical presentation in adolescence (e.g., less hyperactivity, but continued physical restlessness, talkativeness, and problems with behavioral regulation). Go over the main aspects of establishing the diagnosis, with emphasis on the developmental deviance of symptoms. Emphasize the 3–5% prevalence rate. Briefly cover comorbidity—behavioral, academic, emotional, social, and so forth. Also describe how ADHD can affect parental and family functioning. Discuss in more detail the situational variability of ADHD symptoms, that ADHD is not an either–or, all-or-none phenomenon. Its symptoms appear as a function of situational demands, such as whether a situation is boring or interesting, whether the group is large or small, how much feedback the teen gets, and so on. Provide examples to illustrate these points. Briefly discuss etiology, with an emphasis on ADHD being primarily an inborn, biological condition that is hereditary in nature, with far fewer ADHD children having any history of prenatal complications, environmental toxins, or head injury. Also emphasize that ADHD is not caused by diet, family stress, or chaotic home environments. If time permits, review the following:

- The multimodal assessment process.
- The concept of multimodal treatment and the standard treatments for ADHD, as well as treatments that have no research to support their use.
- Medicatons for ADHD, particularly the stimulants.

## Overview of the Disruptive Behavior Disorders

If the teen has not been diagnosed with ADHD, review with the parents the nature of ODD and CD. It will be helpful to parents if you emphasize the role of temperamental factors (such as an inborn predisposition to irritability or aggression) as well as the heritability of these factors (placing parents at greater risk for being irritable or aggression with their child). Invite the parents to describe the behaviors that their teen has displayed that led to the ODD or CD diagnosis, and help parents understand exactly which behaviors are involved with making the diagnostic decision. Parents might also benefit from understanding the distinction between childhood and adolescent onset of the behaviors. It would also be helpful to review the nature of any comorbid conditions such as dysthymia or learning disabilities. (*Note:* Many of the teens we have seen in our program use marijuana or alcohol recreationally. This is clearly a problem to be addressed. However, if the teen is actively engaged in some type of substance abuse that is clearly having a negative impact on their day-to-day functioning, he/she should be in treatment to address the abuse *first*, before enrolling in this treatment program.)

## Common Family Reactions

Clearly there has been a significant amount of material to cover thus far. You need to be stimulating and engaging in these sessions, for if you are too laid-back and reflective, you run the danger of the family getting bored, floundering, and even dropping out. If the teenager has been diagnosed with ADHD, there is a one in four chance that one of the parents will also have similar characteristics (e.g., disorganization, procrastination, distractibility, etc.). The clinician must beware of overinterpreting lateness, missed appointments, or incomplete homework. Ignore the disorganization, be forgiving, and keep a disability perspective. Don't hesitate to work aggressively to keep families coming in.

## Homework

Parents can be instructed to watch the videos on ADHD and ODD (Barkley, 1992a, 1992b, 1997c, 1997d).

# Principles of Behavior Management

## *Goals*

1. To educate parents concerning the causes of teenagers' defiant behavior.

2. To encourage parents to identify the causes of or contributors to defiant behavior that exist in their family.

3. To urge parents to begin to remedy the causes of defiance that can be rectified within their family.

## *Materials Required*

- Parent Handouts for Step 2

    Principles of Behavior Management
    Coercive Behavior Cycle

## *Session Outline*

- Review parents' reaction to the videos.
- Complete the ADHD overview as needed.
- Introduce the four-factor model of teen misbehavior.
- Discuss basic principles of behavior management.
- Describe the coercive behavior cycle.

## *Homework*

- Parents observe and analyze their parenting style in the context of the topics discussed.

This session begins with a review of the parents' reaction to the videos. You can also answer questions and clarify parents' understanding of ADHD if that is relevant.

# A Model for Understanding Teen Misbehavior

Review the model of four possible factors that contribute the teenager's behavior problem, as outlined below. Emphasize that there are many theoretical models "on the market," but for the duration of this program you are asking parents to view their family through the perspective of this model. At the end of the program, they are free to make their own decision about the model's utility.

## The Teen's Psychological Characteristics

The first factor that would contribute to the perception that the teenager has a behavior problem is *teen characteristics*. These are the inborn or otherwise biologically based characteristics that the teen, let's say a boy, carries with him into his interactions with the world. These are *not* learned behaviors. As an example, have the parents reflect on their experiences with their children as infants (or other peoples' infants if they have only one child). Can they agree that not all infants are alike? Some infants are easily soothed, settle quickly into a schedule, and are able to entertain themselves for long periods of time. Other infants are fussy, quick to startle, and display difficulty adjusting to a regular schedule. These are temperamental characteristics that the infant was born with—"neurologically hardwired," so to speak—not the result of how expertly they are cared for. Infants, in other words, are not "blank slates" on which the script of experience will be written. They bring characteristics into the world with them that will make them more or less easy to care for, more or less likely to be viewed as a "problem."

You can also ask parents to consider what they have learned about ADHD. It is an inborn, biologically based developmental disorder that creates the tendency to be overactive, impulsive, and disinhibited. How likely is it that these characteristics in and of themselves will be perceived as a behavior problem? Obviously, quite likely!

Their teen, let's say a girl, also carries within her another characteristic that is simply a biological aspect of who she is, at least for the near future, and that is her age. Being an adolescent in and of itself (at least in Western cultures) may be perceived as a behavioral problem. There are normal processes that all adolescents are expected to go through: becoming more *independent*, developing an *identity* independent of their parents, and preparing themselves for ultimately *separating* from their family. Most parents of teenagers will agree that there is a certain amount of behavioral upheaval that is inevitable during the adolescent years.

## The Parents' Characteristics

The second factor that can contribute to the perception of a behavior problem in the teenager is *parent characteristics*. Parents are also human and may have temperamental or physical characteristics that make it more likely that they will have difficulty with the teen's behavior. For example, a parent who is in chronic pain because of a back injury is going to have less energy and patience to cope with an active, impulsive teen than the parent who does not suffer physical pain. Likewise, the parent who has a psychiatric problem, such as chronic anxiety, will also have less energy and patience than the parent who does not. Parents may also have personality characteristics that are not an optimal "fit" with a teen diagnosed with ODD or ADHD. For example, the parent who is compulsively neat and organized may be far quicker to view the ODD or ADHD teen as a behavior problem than the parent who is more laid-back and less organized.

One particular characteristic of some parents that is especially significant is the presence of ADHD in the parent. If the ODD or ADHD teen is by definition hot tempered, and the parent with ADHD is also hot tempered, the potential for conflict between the two may be far greater than it would be if the parent did not have ADHD.

Parents should be encouraged to discuss their insights into how they may be contributing to behavior problems with their teen.

## Family Stress

The third factor that contributes to the perception of behavioral difficulties is *family stress*. This is a multifaceted concept that can have an impact in a variety of ways. One or both parents may be under stress for a variety of reasons (illness or death of an important family member, legal or financial problems, marital conflict, job problems, etc.). Under the influence of this stress, the parent may become less patient, less tolerant of minor misbehaviors, and quicker to be punitive, leading to increased conflict with the teen. Or, conversely, the parent may be more distracted, withdrawn, and less consistent in implementing common household rules, allowing the teen to "get away with murder" and increasing the likelihood that the teen will be oppositional when the parent eventually returns to enforcing the rules.

In both of these examples, the teen may not even be aware of the exact nature of the stress the parent is under. However, it is critical for parents to understand that teens themselves can also experience stress. This might be "bad" stress, such as getting a failure warning from school, being threatened or bullied by others, or losing a job. Teens can also experience "good" stress, or excitement, over such things as being invited to a party, anticipating school vacation, or getting their driver's license. Ask any teacher what it is like to manage a class the week before Christmas, and you will hear about the impact of excitement on behavior. For the teen with ADHD, who by definition has less internal ability to regulate his behavior than his peers, the impact of either good or bad stress is inevitable: his behavior is going to begin to unravel, becoming more erratic and more impulsive.

## Parenting Style

From the point of view of this theoretical model, the three factors above are not going to be the targets for change. ADHD, for example, is an inborn biological condition for which there is no cure. Parents may choose to address their own characteristics, but that is up to them. And no one has successfully come up with a cure for stress. It is the fourth factor over which we have the greatest control and that will be the focus of the remainder of the program, and that is *parenting style*. Parenting style refers to what parents do in response to their child's behavior, that is, how they handle it. Although parenting style does not cause ADHD, there are some parenting styles that can increase the likelihood of the disruptive behavior disorders, and some that decrease their likelihood. While parenting style does not completely eliminate the impact of the first three factors, it can act as a buffer to mitigate their impact, or a sieve through which the other three factors must be filtered before we ultimately see the child's *behavior*.

# Principles of Behavior Management

This leads us to the topic of behavior management. Ask parents if they have any experience with behavior modification. Tell them that even if they are not familiar with the term, they will be familiar with the concepts. For example, the use of rewards and punishment is part of behavior modification. Explain that behavior modification is very down to earth, rooted in common sense, and—the reason it is the cornerstone of this program—uniquely well-suited to meet the needs of a child with disruptive behavior problems or ADHD.

Use the ABC's of Behavioral Management (in the first parent handout) as a visual aid. Explain that there are two ways to influence or change $B$ (behavior). $A$ formally refers to the "antecedents" of behavior: the cues or triggering events that occur before behavior takes place. For most parents, a more understandable term is "anticipating" behavior before it happens. $C$ refers to the use of "consequences" after the behavior happens. If we put all our energy into $A$ and $C$, $B$ will fall into place.

Provide a simple example of anticipating behavior as a way of changing behavior. One example readily understandable to parents is the common toddler behavior of putting everything into the mouth. Imagine that you have cleaning fluids under your sink. Do you wait for the behavior to happen and then punish it? Certainly not. You anticipate the behavior and shift circumstances around in such a way that the behavior cannot just happen (e.g., adding childproof locks, moving things to a high shelf). *That's* behavior modification! Provide an example of a positive behavior: We want Johnny to complete his worksheet in class. We know that when he sits next to Billy, nothing gets done, but when he sits next to Bobby and Jimmy, he is able to stay on task. Therefore, we anticipate that behavior and make it more likely that it will happen by sitting him next to Bobby and Jimmy.

Anticipating behavior requires forethought and the use of previous experience to predict the future. Whenever parents can do this, it's like money in the bank. However, often behavior cannot be anticipated, and parents must deal with behaviors after they have taken place.

Research on behavior modification tells us that *positive consequences* make it more likely that a behavior will happen again, and *negative consequences* make it less likely that a behavior will happen again. Although this makes sense, parents may not be aware that they are sometimes inadvertently rewarding a negative behavior, making it more likely that it will happen again, or punishing a positive behavior, making it less likely that it will happen again. We will address those problems later in this program. For now, let's assume that the parents of the defiant teen have tried rewards and punishments and feel frustrated and discouraged that they haven't worked. Why not? Because for the defiant or ADHD teen, the connection between their *B*ehavior and the *C*onsequence for their behavior is very easily lost. Once lost, even the most sophisticated behavior-modification system is not going to change behavior. Therefore, we have to work diligently to keep that connection crystal clear. To do so, three concepts must be put into place.

Be **specific**. For example, the parent says to the teen, let's say a boy, "Clean your room." Fifteen minutes later, the parent looks into the room and notices that the bed isn't made. The parent says to the teen, who is playing a video game, "I thought I told you to clean your room!" The teen looks up at the hamper where he stuffed all his dirty clothes and says, "But I did clean my room." The parent responds, "But you didn't make your bed," and the teen says, "But you didn't ask me to make my bed." And he's right!

A parent may say at this point that every day of his life the teen has had to make his bed, so this isn't a very convincing example. But let's examine what happened. If the teen has ADHD, he may have gone to his room with good intentions and put the dirty clothes into the hamper. But then his eye is caught by the screen saver on his computer and he is drawn off-task by the allure of a far more interesting activity. Alternatively, the ODD teen may quite manipulatively say to himself, "I put the clothes in the hamper, that's good enough." A more specific request ("Make your bed" rather than "Clean your room") increases the likelihood that the teen will follow through.

Similarly, parents are often extremely vague about consequences, such as "Clean your room or you'll be in big trouble." This type of vague threat is probably so familiar to the teen that he can quite accurately predict that it will amount to almost nothing, and therefore it has no influence on his behavior. "Make your bed and you can use the telephone; if you do not make your bed by 8 A.M., you will lose telephone privileges for the rest of the day" is a very specific consequence.

It is very important to emphasize to parents: Don't be vague. Don't be general. Be specific.

The next key component in keeping the connection between behavior and consequences clear is to be **immediate**. For each minute that passes between the teen's behavior and the consequence imposed by the parent, the connection becomes weaker and the consequence becomes less powerful. This is true even for positive consequences. Of course it is not always realistic to provide a consequence immediately (and it is certainly true that a delayed consequence is better than no consequence at all). Parents of a teen diagnosed with ADHD must understand the difficulty with time perception that individuals with ADHD experience. For teens with ADHD, the world they live in is *now*. They do not think ahead or reflect on the past unless assisted and guided to do so. This is the nature of their disability. Therefore, for consequences, either positive or negative, to have a powerful influence on their behavior, they must also occur *now*.

The final concept that keeps the connection between behavior and consequences clear is to be **consistent**. Most teens can figure out that there are different rules for Mom in a good mood, Mom in a bad mood, Mom when Dad is around, Dad when Mom isn't around, and so forth, and they will abide by the rules accordingly. But for defiant or ADHD teens, who have trouble internalizing and following rules anyway, the more variable the rules, the more likely it is that the teen will fail. When there is one set of rules, for Mom and Dad, for good mood and bad mood, and so on, it increases the likelihood that the teen will be able to comply. Similarly, when the consequence is consistent (e.g., you *never* get dessert if you don't eat your vegetables), the teen is more likely to be influenced by that consequence.

No parent is 100% specific, immediate, or consistent. It is not humanly possible. Our goal in this program is simply to move parents in that direction.

Parents also need to be cognizant of the qualities of consequences that will make them more or less effective. First, consequences need to be **meaningful**, that is, meaningful to the teen. Many parents are frustrated, for example, that their ADHD teen is not motivated by "pride in accomplishment," "a sense of responsibility," or "respect for elders." These are weak goals—they do not result in an immediate, positive reward. Parents will do well to accept the fact that their ADHD teen is far more likely to be motivated by tangible, exciting, fun, stimulating consequences than by long-term, intangible ones.

Consequences for defiant or ADHD teens also work best when they are **frequent**. Parents must understand that "consequences" encompass words of praise, a smile, a thumbs-up, a reprimand, or a hug. Individuals with ADHD in particular thrive on frequent feedback. It keeps them on track, like the automatic pilot in a jet plane. A "patter" of comments and interaction throughout the day will assist the teen with ADHD to regulate his behavior.

Lastly, consequences need to be **well balanced**. If the number of negative consequences that the teen receives far outweighs the number of positive consequences, he will become demoralized and we will lose his motivation. This issue is so important that it will form the basis of our first specific exercise, discussed in Step 3.

## The Coercive Behavior Cycle

The last topic to be covered in this session refers back to an earlier comment about how parents sometimes inadvertently reward a negative behavior, strange as that may sound. It is best to give parents a common example of this behavior so they can determine whether it is relevant in their home:

Imagine it is a typical day in the life of a family with a defiant teen, let's say a girl. The parent makes a request, such as "Take out the trash." If it is a particularly good day, the teen complies and life goes on. (Give the handout for this session to the parent and describe the coercive cycle.)

$$\text{Request} \rightarrow \text{Compliance}$$

But if it truly is a typical day, the task does not get done (the teen is busy, she'll get to it later, etc.), and the request is repeated several times.

$$\text{Request} \rightarrow \text{Noncompliance}$$

After a while, the parent will probably begin to get irritated and will escalate the request, that is, make a few threats, raise his/her voice, assume an ugly look on his/her face. In response, the teen may comply or she may escalate her refusal, shout at the parent, slam the door, swear, and so on. This can go around until everyone is good and angry:

$$\text{Request!!} \rightarrow \text{Noncompliance!!!}$$

At this point one of two things is likely to happen. Either the parent will *force* the teen to comply, through physical intimidation. Or, if the parent is tired, if they just can't deal with it anymore, they will *give up.*

Ask parents if they have ever given up and done the task themselves. They are quite likely to answer in the affirmative. Explain to them that for the teen, this scenario is like gambling: the teen knows that when the parent makes a request, the odds are in his favor that if he resists, he will not have to comply. *"Noncompliance"* is the negative behavior—"give up" is the reward.

Tell parents that the first thing that they must do in this program is to break this cycle. They must no longer "give up." If they make a request, the teen must either comply or experience a negative consequence. Therefore, parents must think before they ask the teen to do something: "Do I have the energy to follow through, do I have a consequence planned, should I make a smaller request so I can handle the situation more easily?" For this early part of the program, parents may decide simply not to make any requests at all until they learn how to use consequences appropriately. This is acceptable.

## Common Family Reactions

A great wealth of material is covered in this session. Watch for parents becoming overwhelmed. If you take it slow and steady, avoid psychological jargon, and ask them to give you examples, their understanding will become a source of empowerment as they confront the coercive teen. Be sure to remind parents to anticipate an escalation in the teen's negative reactions to the attempts by parents to reassert control over his/her behavior. Parents should interpret this not as a sign of failure, but as a sign of potential success. If parents persist in their new parenting style, the teen's resistance will eventually decrease.

## Homework

Parents should be instructed to observe and analyze their parenting style in the context of the issues discussed during this session. For example, they can experiment with being more specific, can make a list of consequences that are meaningful to the teen, or can try more frequent feedback. Finally, instruct them that they are not to "give up" anymore.

# Developing Positive Attention

## _Goals_

1. To educate parents about how the style of their interactions with their teen greatly affects the teen's motivation to work for them.

2. To train parents in methods of attending to positive teen behavior while ignoring minor misbehaviors.

3. To begin establishing a more positive interaction pattern between parent and teen through these positive attending skills.

## _Materials Required_

- Parent Handout for Step 3

    Paying Attention to Your Teen's Good Behavior

## _Session Outline_

- Address carry-over concerns from Sessions 1 and 2.
- Review homework.

    Parental attempts to view family life through the four-factor model
    Parental attempts to utilize the principles of behavior management

- Introduce the rationale for developing positive attending skills.
- Discuss importance of quality of attention to people.
- Present "worst" versus "best" supervisor vignette.
- Extend discussion to how parents attend to problem teen.
- Review the mechanics of conducting positive, one-on-one time with the teen.

- Review mechanics of ignoring minor misbehaviors.
- Determine when one-on-one time will be done at home.

*Homework*

- Each parent practices positive, one-on-one time with the teen two to three times over the coming week.

This session begins with a brief review of Sessions 1 and 2. Answer any questions parents may have about ODD or ADHD (e.g., definition, etiology, diagnostic evaluation, cormorbidity, effective treatments). Avoid lengthy discussions about school-related problems at this point, deferring to later sessions. Briefly highlight the main points: ADHD is primarily an inborn, biological, developmental delay; defiant teenagers, particularly those diagnosed with ADHD, are at risk for parent–child conflict, which can be exacerbated by various child, parent, stress, and parenting-style characteristics. We will now begin to work on developing a parenting style that will be the best possible fit for a defiant teen.

## The Rationale for Developing Positive Attending Skills

Discuss the importance of beginning with the positive attending skills. There are three reasons why we begin the program with the positive strategies. First, in many families who have experienced months or years of misbehavior, problems, frustration, punishment, and the like, the overall family atmosphere becomes very negative. The teen may feel that he/she is always in trouble; the parents may feel depressed and demoralized because all they do is "yell" at their child. We start with the positives in order to lighten the tone and help everyone feel more optimistic.

Second, exclusive use of negative strategies (e.g., punishment), even if they are excellent strategies, will not be sufficient to turn the situation around. Most of the families who come into the clinic will be using reasonable (albeit inconsistent) forms of punishment (we see very little in the way of unusual or exotic punishments) and will see no improvement in their teen's behavior. Tell the parents that their own personal experience simply confirms what research has been telling us all along: exclusive and inconsistent use of punishment is insufficient. If they add positive strategies and become more consistent, the very same punishment strategies will become much more effective.

Finally, we start with the positive strategies in order to strike a balance between the number of positive interactions and the number of negative interactions the parents have with their child over the course of the day. For a family with a child without behavior problems, throughout the day there may be a word of praise here, a smile and a hug there, as well as a reprimand here, a criticism there. Spontaneously, without anyone really having to think about it, the situation balances out. For the family with a defiant teen, the number of reprimands and criticisms may be very high, while the opportunities for positive comments may seem almost nonexistent. In the face of this unbalanced situation, the teen has little motivation to even try to improve his/her behavior (and if this is true at home, it is even more true in a classroom). We need to correct the imbalance *not* by dramatically reducing the negatives; we may reduce them a little, but it would be unrealistic to reduce them more since the teen does misbehave and does require negative feedback. What we will do instead is dramatically increase the positives. It will seem awkward and almost artificial at first, but it is crucial to make sure that some sort of positive interaction is happening at least as many times (if not more) than negative interaction. Parents need to understand and accept that this means they will be interacting with their teen much more frequently throughout the course of the day than would the parent of a nondefiant teen—this is important because of the need for more externalized methods for regulating behavior.

## "Pay Positive Attention"

Tell parents that the first strategy they will be practicing is to "pay positive attention." Everyone appreciates positive attention, including teenagers. A nice way to illustrate this is to have parents think back over their own experiences and recall their most favorite boss, supervisor, or teacher, as well as their least favorite. When each parent has successfully recalled two specific individuals (without naming names!), ask them to start by describing the least favorite: What was that person like, what did they say, what did they do—what made them the least favorite supervisor. Make a list of attributes on a piece of paper or whiteboard, encouraging parents to be specific and descriptive (this is fun to do with a group of parents). Do the same with the most favorite supervisor. Then summarize the two lists and ask parents to describe what it felt like to work for these two individuals: Did it affect their feelings about their job, did it affect their motivation? Parents will inevitably tell you "Yes." Ask parents now to think of these two characters at two ends of a continuum, and say, "Now imagine the world of adults from your child's point of view. Where would various people fall on this continuum? Where would you fall?" The more an adult falls toward the least favorite supervisor end of the continuum, the less likely it is that the teen will be interested or motivated to please that person, to go the "extra mile," so to speak, when anything is demanded of the teen. Many parents of defiant teens have slid, over the years, against their best intentions, toward that least favorite supervisor role. The goal of this first exercise is to take parents, wherever they happen to fall on the continuum, and move them toward the most favorite supervisor end. That way they are more likely to be able to inspire their teen to want to please them.

### Spend One-On-One Time

The exercise for parents to pay positive attention to their teen is called "one-on-one time." There are several ways of going about this exercise, but the basic premise is always the same: one parent spends at least 10–15 minutes alone with the teen, during which time the teen does something that he enjoys doing, and the parent refrains from asking questions or giving commands, and makes only positive or neutral, descriptive comments instead. Emphasize to the parent that this is easier said than done. If you have ever tried to spend 15 minutes with a child without asking any questions, you will understand.

*Point One:* The teen is doing something he enjoys doing. One possibility is to simply tell the teen that you have 15 minutes to spare and you would like to do something with him— what would he like to do? Many teens, especially the younger ones, can be surprisingly enthusiastic about this. They get to chose the activity, as long as it is "within reason," that is, not a normally forbidden activity or one that is too time-consuming or expensive. Examples including playing a video game, cooking, shooting hoops, working in the woodshop, and the like.

Another possibility is for the parent simply to wait for a time when the teen is already engaged in an activity on his own that lends itself to this exercise, and then to "hang around" for a while, making positive comments. This approach is especially appropriate for teens who are suspicious, cynical, or disinterested in spending time with a parent. Alternatively, the time spent driving to the store, a doctor's appointment, and so forth, if it is in the spirit of this exercise, could be considered one-on-one time.

*Point Two:* The parent asks no questions, makes no corrections, gives no instructions or directions. The parent must temporarily drop the role of "teacher" and adopt a nonjudgmental, positive stance. Questions *direct* the conversation, and therefore are eliminated so that the teen can direct the interaction. Corrections, directions, and instructions are all judgmental and are therefore eliminated in the service of creating a brief period of nonjudgmental observations.

*Point Three:* The parent makes either positive comments or neutral, descriptive comments. Parents don't have to be "phony" here. They can genuinely look for the opportunity to say something positive ("Nice job," "I like the way you did that"). But they should not lie— they can always be purely descriptive ("That music has both guitars and a keyboard"). One approach is to describe the action like a sports commentator. Another approach is to be a "reflective listener."

## Ignore Minor Misbehavior

If during the exercise the teen begins to do something that the parent feels is annoying, he/she needs to decide if it is a minor misbehavior (i.e., irritating but not disrespectful or a violation of a household rule) or more serious. If the behavior is minor, the parent briefly turns away and stops talking (ignores) until the behavior stops, even for a split second, and then the parent makes a positive comment. If the behavior escalates into a more major problem, then the parent stops the exercise and corrects the behavior.

One-on-one time is not used as a reward. The teen does not earn it for good behavior, or lose it for bad behavior. The parent should look for an appropriate opportunity to spend one-on-one time with the teen, apart from times when he/she is being punished for some other problem.

Problem-solve in advance with parents issues such as what to do with other siblings, how to create time for the exercise when schedules are extremely busy, or how to predict what the teen might chose to do.

## Common Family Reactions

Many parents are convinced that the last thing their teenager wants to do is spend time with them. You should not try to change their minds directly, but simply ask them to agree that for the time they are in this program they will try to practice each assignment in good faith. At the end of the program, they are free to make their own more informed decision about the utility of each exercise.

The most common family reaction is to return to the next session reporting that "it was a busy week" and therefore they had no time to practice. Be sympathetic but firm about the importance of creating even a few minutes of space for the exercise, and emphasize the potential benefits: a more positive relationship with the teen and the teen's improved self-esteem.

## Homework

Give parents the handout. Ask each parent to engage in one-on-one time daily if possible, but at least two or three times before the next session.

# Developing Parental Attending Skills

## Goals

1. To train parents to use effective attending skills that will increase immediate teen compliance with commands.
2. To increase parents' use of effective attending skills in the absence of the teen's common misbehaviors.
3. To increase the effectiveness of parental commands in eliciting teen compliance.

## Materials Required

- Parent Handout for Step 4

    How to Give Effective Commands

## Session Outline

- Review implementation of one-on-one time, positive attending, and ignoring.
- Discuss extension of positive attending and ignoring to other areas.

    Spontaneous compliance
    Absence of common misbehaviors

- Teach parents ways of issuing effective commands.

## Homework

- Practice praising teen for the absence of common misbehaviors.
- Practice praising teen for spontaneous compliance.
- Practice giving effective commands.

Review implementation of one-on-one time. Have parents describe their use of positive attending skills in activities chosen by the teen or in spontaneous situations. Also review the use of ignoring minor misbehaviors. Review and discuss the teen's reaction. Refine the implementation of Session 3 strategies as needed.

Be sure to practice what you preach: Praise parents liberally if they performed the exercise. If they did not, clarify the importance of practicing and reassign the exercise as homework for the remainder of the program.

Since parents have now had the opportunity to experience the use of nonjudgmental positive attention, we will begin to use that positive attention *contingently*, that is, as a consequence for appropriate behaviors. But we will start out with easily attainable goals and save the more challenging behaviors for the next session. Essentially, the theme for Session 4 is to learn how to *catch the teen being good*. Parents will be instructed in how to set their teen up to succeed, so that both the teen and they will have opportunities to experience behavioral success. This will be accomplished by practicing two simple, brief exercises. As neither of the exercises is particularly time-consuming, parents should continue to practice one-on-one time as well.

## Praise for the Absence of Common Misbehaviors

The first exercise is to increase the use of praise for the *absence of common misbehaviors*. Explain to parents that all teenagers can be disruptive at times. However, because defiant teens, particularly those with ADHD, are impulsive and impatient by nature, they have even more trouble waiting for things. Therefore, these teens frequently interrupt parents when they're busy. They are also more active and fidgety than other teens, so they often engage in irritating behaviors such as rapping on the table with their silverware. In addition, they are deficient in their ability to regulate their behavior and frequently violate minor household rules, such as talking with their mouths full.

Have parents describe common misbehaviors in the home, and ask how they've handled one particular situation (typically it will be either by reprimanding or by redirecting the teen). Note that this has not corrected the problem and ask the parents if they can think of reasons why this approach has not worked (e.g., an imbalance of positive and negative feedback). Now ask them to imagine the same scenario, but this time the teen's irritating behavior does not occur for some reason. What would they do? The answer will probably be "nothing." Perhaps the parents take the "let sleeping dogs lie" philosophy, or perhaps they take the absence of misbehavior for granted. In either case, the result is that the parent "ignores" the positive behavior (i.e., the absence of the misbehavior).

Against this backdrop, predict that the opposite of what they have been doing will work better. They should target one or two common minor misbehaviors, and over the following week go out of their way to praise the teen when the behavior does not occur in a situation where they would normally expect it. Ask parents to put this strategy to the test, emphasizing that the effects will be gradual but real. They should also continue to increase the amount of praise occurring in the household.

## Praise for Spontaneous Compliance

The second exercise utilizes praise for *spontaneous compliance*. Ask parents to estimate the following: For every 100 times they issue a command and the teen does not comply, how often do they attend negatively? For every 100 times they issue a command and the teen does comply, how often do they attend positively? Many parents will tell you that the teen never complies. You should then explain that not all commands are created equal. "Make your bed" is a command, but so is "Pass me a tissue" or "Get yourself a soda." Some commands are much more attractive or less onerous than others. It is the *process* that we emphasize in this exercise: parent issues a command, teen complies, parent praises. The *content* of the command should set the teen up to succeed. Thus, for this exercise, parents should ask the teen to do something simple or attractive at least once a day and then go out of their way to praise the teen's compliance. Give many examples, and ask parents to describe what sorts of requests they will make (e.g., passing the salt, turning on a favorite TV program, holding the door, getting a piece of cake, etc.).

## Effective Commands

Go over strategies for giving commands more effectively. Parents first need to consider their own *intent* when they make a command: Do they really mean it seriously? Do they have the time and energy to follow through and make sure the command is followed? Is there a consequence already thought out for possible noncompliance? If any of these answers are "No," the parent should not issue the command. If all the answers are "Yes," then the parent should communicate their intent through tone of voice and body language.

Parents should avoid ambiguity when issuing commands. For example, many parents phrase commands as questions—"Do you want to do your homework now?"—which implies that the teen has a choice. If in fact the teen does have a choice, then phrasing in this fashion is fine. But if there is no choice, then this phrasing is ambiguous, and will be particularly confusing for an ADHD teen. Likewise, parents should not respond to compliance with gratitude, as if somehow the teen has done them a favor (e.g., "Thank you for doing your homework"). Praise ("Great job getting that homework done!") is the appropriate response. In addition, defiant teens benefit from being told *what to do* rather than *what not to do*. In a very face-saving way, it gives them information about what their next step should be, which might otherwise not occur to them spontaneously (e.g., "Put your sneakers in the closet" instead of "Don't leave your sneakers in the middle of the living room").

In giving commands, parents of teens with ADHD must never forget that commands should not be issued when there are competing distractions going on, such as the TV or the stereo. Likewise, multistep commands may need to be broken down into single steps, or written lists may be used. Finally, any command that involves the concept of time (e.g., "Be ready by 5 P.M." or "You have 15 minutes to clean your room") may be extremely challenging for the teen with ADHD. Use aids to assist the teen with time, such as a digital clock or a timer, or simply put as many commands as possible in the context of "now."

## Common Family Reactions

Families do not always grasp the significance of Session 4. In essence, however, once they find themselves consistently practicing the concepts described in this session, they will truly be "proactive parents," not "reactive parents": They are creating a balance between the positive and negative interactions they have with their teen. In addition, the household is being flooded with positive feedback. Finally, the feedback is increasingly geared to the information processing style of an individual with ADHD.

## Homework

Give parents the handout. Ask them to practice each of the two exercises daily, and to begin to utilize effective commands. Set realistic expectations for change. Remind them to call you for assistance if necessary.

# Establishing a Behavioral Contract

## *Goals*

1. To establish a formal system that makes teen privileges contingent upon teen compliance. This is achieved by implementing either a behavioral contract or a point system.

2. To increase parental attention to and reinforcement of teen compliance and appropriate social conduct.

3. To decrease arbitrariness in parental administration of child privileges.

## *Materials Required*

- Parent Handouts for Step 5

    Sample Behavioral Contract
    The Home Point System

## *Session Outline*

- Review parental extension of positive attending and ignoring skills to areas discussed in Session 4. Also review efforts to improve how commands are given.

- Set up a home-based behavioral contract or point system.

## *Homework*

- Initiate use of the point system or a behavioral contract.

Review homework on attending skills. Have parents describe their attempts to praise the teen in the absence of misbehavior and to increase their praise for spontaneous compliance. Also have parents describe their attempts to give commands more effectively. Ask them to describe the teen's response to these strategies. Be sure to commend parents for practicing and make corrections in their implementation as needed. If parents did not practice, clarify why and remind them of the importance of practicing what they learn. Reassign Session 4 homework if necessary.

## The Contingency-Management System

Provide parents with the rationale behind setting up a "contingency-management system." For example, many teens are saturated with material goods: electronic equipment, sporting goods, telephone, possibly even a car. A typical teenager's room might look like an annex of a department store. Not only do many parents feel obligated to make these material goods available to their children, but most teens take these things for granted and assume that they are "rights." When the teen misbehaves, parents take things away, but this often does not work because the teen has many other fun things to do. Conversely, when parents try to use rewards to promote good behavior, it may not work because the teen does not need this extra thing—he/she has enough already. Inherent in this scenario is that the teen is in control of these things most of the time, not parents; parents only step in when misbehavior occurs, by taking things away. In other words, it is a system of parenting in which parents primarily attend to the teen when negative behavior occurs.

Contrast this to the situation where all fun things are defined as "privileges" that the teen must earn through the display of appropriate behavior. Ask parents to reflect on their own childhoods: Are there things that their child takes for granted that they themselves clearly viewed as a privilege when they were growing up? A "right" is yours no matter what (e.g., food, clothing, safety—these are state-defined rights). Parents may also decide that something is their teen's "right," such as access to the bike he/she bought with money from his/her birthday. In contrast, a "privilege" is something you earn, and by definition is under parental control.

Parents will probably need help understanding that they do in fact have control over many things in their teen's life, such as the telephone (if they pay the bill) or the TV or computer (if they bought the machine or pay the electricity bill). Parents need to be encouraged to "empower" themselves by identifying where they have control and then using it positively. Discuss with parents the idea that there is a "motivation" deficit in defiant teens, wherein they cannot persist in goal-directed, task-oriented behaviors, such as chores or tasks, without consequences to keep them motivated. Compared to normal teenagers, they require more salient or powerful consequences to achieve compliance. As a result, parents must accept the idea that they may have to promise more tangible, salient, and material reinforcers to get defiant teens to comply with rules that would not be required for normal teens. Be prepared to address concerns about bribery, becoming materialistic, the loss of the intrinsic appeal of work, and so forth. Research, for example, suggests that social reinforcement alone does not work as well for children with ADHD. Lacking internal controls for self-regulation, they require more external controls and/or motivation to keep their behavior on task and to comply with parental expectations. They do not routinely stop and think about the consequences of their behavior *before* they act. They also require more specific, frequent, immediate, and consistent feedback, as well as more tangible or materialistic rewards.

## Behavioral Contracts

If the teen is over the age of 14, set up a behavioral contract system. First, have parents write down the requests or chores they routinely ask of the teen that do not always get done right away. These should be fairly specific items which, when requested, must be done immediately, allowing parents to respond immediately (e.g., starting homework, making bed, etc.). They should not list "don't behaviors" (e.g., don't swear, don't hit siblings, etc.); these will be addressed later. Once the list is created, have parents rank order the requests based on how difficult it is for the teen to comply, in terms of time, effort, and likelihood of compliance. Next have parents construct a list of "privileges," those items or activities that are highly desirable to the teen (preferably on a daily basis) and are under parental control. Privileges should be very specific (e.g., 1 hour of TV time).

For the first behavioral contract, have the parents choose a request of relatively low difficulty and a privilege of moderate value to the teen. Instruct parents to inform the teen that for the following week, he/she will not have access to the privilege unless and until the request is completed. This instruction should be written in the form of a contract that both parents (and usually the teen) initial; the teen receives a copy. Provide parents with blank copies of the behavioral contract handout for use at home.

> *I, Bobby Jones, agree that I will make my bed each weekday morning before I leave for school. If my bed is made, I can use the telephone after school. If my bed is not made, I cannot use the telephone for the rest of the day.*

## The Point System

If the teen is 13 years old or is a somewhat less mature older teen, parents should set up a home point system. In this system, each request is assigned a point value, depending on how hard it is for the teen to accomplish the task (use a point spread from 100 to 1,000 in increments of 100). Privileges are also assigned points depending on how attractive they are (make sure that the privilege list has a mixture of daily and weekly privileges). Of the total value of the request list, one half to two thirds should be equivalent to the value of all the daily privileges; one half to one third times five (for five weekdays) should be equivalent to the total value of the weekly privileges. Parents should explain to the teen that whenever he/she does anything on the request list the first time he/she is asked, the appropriate number of points will be entered into his/her "checkbook" (the register portion of a checkbook, where a running balance is kept). When he/she wants something on the privilege list, the appropriate number of points will be deducted from his/her running balance. The teen cannot do anything on the privilege list unless he/she has enough points and pays for the privilege *before* actually doing it; in other words, no credit is allowed. Parents are the only ones who handle the checkbook, but the teen is allowed to see it anytime that he/she wants to see how many points are available.

Parents should be informed that many teens will resist the point system at first, and may even threaten to quit participating after a day or two. Once presented, however, the program must be implemented regardless of how much resistance the teen displays. The teen's resistance is simply an attempt to keep the old system in place, which is counterproductive to the family. If parents clearly communicate their conviction to use the program, the resistance will eventually dissipate. If parents are not willing to hold their ground when the teen resists, they should not start the program until they are ready. Set realistic expectations—the main goal is for parents to alter their parenting style. If the teen's behavior changes, that's a bonus for this week; behavior change may not occur until much later, however. Provide parents with a copy of the handout on the point system and have them read it before leaving so that you can address any questions.

## Common Family Reactions

Parents' most common reaction to setting up a contingency-management system is to overestimate or underestimate the control they can exercise over the teen's privileges. In overestimating, the parents may think they can control access to a privilege when they are not physically in the home. This is a mistake that parents must avoid, since it sets the teen up for dishonesty. If the parent is not physically in the home, or cannot physically remove (or unplug) the privileged item, then they need to view it as out of their control. Conversely, many parents do not know which areas they can control, in great part because the teen has reigned supreme for so long in the home. For example, even if the parent purchased a computer for the teen, the computer is under the control of the parent, not the teen. If the teen needs to be driven to a social gathering, transportation is under the control of the parent, not the teen. When the teen uses the family car, watches the family TV, uses the family telephone, all are under parental control. By exercising their control, parents become empowered to redirect the teen's noncompliant, oppositional behavior in a more positive direction.

## Homework

Parents should either discuss the behavioral contract with the teen and implement it for one week, or review the point system with the teen, making the discussion as positive as possible. Parents should only *dispense* points during the first week; if the request is not followed, the teen simply does not earn that number of points (during the next session, penalties will be described). Have parents bring either the contract or the checkbook register to the next session. Urge them to call for assistance as needed.

# Using Response Cost

*Goal*

- To introduce the use of fines or penalties into home-based contingency management as punishment for noncompliance and unacceptable social conduct.

*Materials Required*

- None

*Session Outline*

- Review implementation of the reward-oriented behavioral contract or point system.
- Add response cost for noncompliance and violation of household rules.

*Homework*

- Begin deducting points or implementing penalties for noncompliance.

Review implementation of the behavioral contract or home-based point system. Have parents describe their implementation of the program with a focus on how comfortable they are with the mechanics of either writing a contract or using the checkbook register. Have parents discuss any problems they experienced defining or choosing privileges, assigning point values, or putting these issues into writing. Review the contract or checkbook register and make adjustments as necessary. Discuss any confrontations with the teen over access to privileges.

If the teen reacted negatively to the contract or point system, explain to parents that the teen may try to coerce them out of continuing this program. Coercion may take the form of arguments, belligerence, or refusal to obey rules of the contract. Make sure that parents understand that they should not give in to coercive attempts, as giving in will reinforce such coercion in the future. Discuss with parents the limits of their own personal control and at what point they would be advised to seek outside assistance from the police, juvenile court, or state department of social services. Advise parents that at no time should they engage in any physical confrontation with the teen, and if they feel that the teen's or their own safety is in danger, they should contact the police.

Be sure to commend parents for practicing the strategies, or get them to clarify why they did not, and then remind them of the importance of home practice. For parents using the point system, remind them of the need to rotate new privileges onto the privilege list periodically to avoid teen boredom with the program.

## Use of Penalties

Give the rationale for penalizing noncompliance with requests or violations of household rules. Remind parents that rewards alone are not enough to maintain appropriate behavior. We generally need to use *penalties* in association with rewards. What is critical, however, is that "the penalty fit the crime." For noncompliance with day-to-day requests to complete chores, or violation of household rules that are not severe in nature, taking privileges or points away is the appropriate response. Grounding is used for more serious problems.

### Behavioral Contracts

For parents using behavioral contracts, identify a "do not" behavior, for example, "Do not hit your brother" or "Do not swear." Next, identify a privilege that is very meaningful to the teen and that the parents could withhold should the need arise. Then write a contract:

> *I, John Smith, agree that I will not swear at my parents. I understand that if I do, I will not get a ride to school in the morning and will have to take the bus.*

Again, parents review the contract with the teen to make sure he understands it, and all initial it.

### The Point System

Parents using the point system should inform the teen that from now on failure to do a chore on the list will lead to an immediate fine/deduction of points. The fine is the amount the teen would have been paid for doing the job. In addition to fines related to chores, have parents create fines for the violation of two of the household rules (e.g., whining, arguing, swearing, taking things without permission, etc.). Determine these point amounts in the session; less severe misbehavior is fined a smaller amount.

Give guidelines for implementing penalty strategies. Parents should discuss these strategies with the teen *before* implementing them. The teen probably will not like the procedure, but they're not supposed to like it. It's intended to be mildly aversive, so as to serve as a reminder to the teen that compliance with requests is more reinforcing than noncompliance. Parents should describe the contract or penalty procedure in a very business-like, matter-of-fact way, pointing out that there is still room for improvement in the teen's behavior and therefore the need for penalties, which will help *remind* him to comply better. To help offset any negative repercussions from using penalties, over the next week parents should go out of their way to catch the teen being good and reward him with praise, "bonus points" (e.g., 100 points), or a spontaneous small reward.

## Common Family Reactions

Many parents assume that their teenager will know exactly what they mean when they identify a household rule like "No talking back." However, these rules are often less specific than they should be. Therefore, the teen may benefit from a 1 week "training period." During this 1 week period, the parent "labels" the misbehavior every time it happens and warns the teen that after the week is over, the behavior will be fined. For example, "That's what I mean by talking back. Starting next Monday you will lose 500 points if you talk back."

Parents may also be vulnerable to "punishment spirals" in which a fine elicits negative affect or coercion from the teen, which the parent then fines again, escalating the negative behavior by the teen, the parent's fines, and so on. The rule for such instances is to fine no more than twice and then redirect the teen to "cool off" away from the situation ("Go to your room," "Sit at the dining room table until you can calm down," etc.). If the teen is unwilling to remove himself, parents should remove themselves from the room so as to terminate the interaction.

Often parents want to use fines for lying, but claim that it is "unfair" to fine the teen for lying when they are not really sure of what happened. Encourage parents to view themselves as the "judge and jury": They may not have witnessed the crime, but they must nonetheless weigh the evidence and pass judgment. It is far better to make it clear to the teen that lying will not be tolerated and perhaps make a mistake in judgment than to allow a teen to lie without consequences. (Parents know their children well and are usually right, but if they find that they have made a mistake, they can simply apologize.) Also, stress that it is the teen's job to remain *above* suspicion, which means that the teen should never give the parent any cause to suspect the teen is lying. Parents should fine based on a suspicion of a lie, for which no real evidence is needed.

Parents should be aware that as they introduce the penalty portion of the program, they may notice that they need to raise their voices or "yell" less frequently. In fact, the program should reduce their stress level because they are planning ahead rather than dealing with each problem reactively as it arises. There is no place in this program for yelling or physical punishment, and it is a great relief to parents to actually be able to *discipline* (i.e., educate) their child rather than simply punish him. If parents are reluctant to use penalties out of concern for the teen's self-esteem, map out the following diagram:

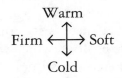

Explain that the emphasis in this program is on "warm" (e.g., positive, loving) and "firm" (e.g., specific, immediate, and consistent). Many parents are afraid of using penalties for fear of being "cold," and they therefore end up being "soft," which allows the further development of coercive behavior in the teen.

## Homework

Implement a new behavioral contract, or introduce penalties to the point system (if parents have not used the point system for at least 1 week, delay introduction of penalties until it has been). Urge parents to call for assistance as needed.

(*Note:* If parents need more time to practice the strategies from Sessions 5 and 6, you may "float" the session on school advocacy [Session 9] into the sequence at any point between Sessions 5 and 10.)

# Completing the Contract/Point System

## *Goal*

- To encourage parents to use a contingency-management approach for any behavior problems their teen displays.

## *Materials Required*

- None

## *Session Outline*

- Review use of behavioral contracts or the point system to date.
- Expand use of behavioral contracts to those teen behaviors of greatest concern to parents.
- Anticipate future problems with the point system.

## *Homework*

- Continue to use the point system or behavioral contracts to address problematic behaviors.

Review in detail the parents' attempts at using response cost for failure to perform chores and for social misconduct. Address any problems that have arisen in implementing the program. Watch for parental escalation of anger during situations in which they fine the teen or take away privileges. Possibly discuss anger-control techniques if escalation has been a problem (e.g., leaving the room, concentrating on being business-like about techniques, asking a spouse to moderate the parent–teen discussion, etc.).

Check with parents on the consistency of the program, especially between parents in their use of the methods. Have parents identify the sources of the inconsistency if this exists (e.g., work schedules, parental philosophy about discipline, etc.). Also, review which parent is carrying the greatest weight in implementing the methods and tracking the behaviors (e.g., who is managing the checkbook register or keeping track of the contracts) in the program. If undue burden is carried by one spouse, discuss this and resolve discrepancies if possible.

For those families using behavioral contracts, review the list of chores and household rules created in Session 5, and determine those three or four tasks most important for the parents to see the teen comply with, as well as an additional household rule if there is another salient one. Write out behavioral contracts for each of these, choosing incentives and penalties that are both meaningful to the teen as well as of reasonable impact (i.e., make sure the penalty fits the crime).

For those families using the point system, emphasize the need to keep the privilege list fresh and meaningful to the teen; otherwise he will no longer be motivated to earn points. Trouble-shoot any problems the parents are having with the mechanics of keeping the checkbook register, stressing the importance of avoiding any teen "tampering" with the amounts entered.

## Common Family Reactions

Some families will report that their teenager responds in a very blasé fashion to penalties or response cost, with comments such as "Go ahead and take it away, I don't care." This response should not be taken as a sign to parents that the program is ineffective. Parents must evaluate for themselves whether (1) the penalty does not have sufficient value to motivate the teen or (2) the penalty has significant value and the teen is using the "go ahead—I don't care" strategy to get parents to back off. Parents know their children, and they can generally judge quite effectively which items or activities are meaningful to the teen. If they truly believe that the penalty matters to the teen, they should simply ignore the "I don't care" statements.

Alternatively, some teens respond to response cost or penalties with coercion in the form of what we call "emotional blackmail": "I hate you," "You're ruining my life," "No one else's parents are as mean as you are," or even "I'm going to report you." Many parents are excruciatingly vulnerable to these sorts of statements and will become concerned or confused about the appropriateness of the penalty. In these situations, if parents know that the penalty they have chosen is fair and just, then they have to run the teen's words through a "translator" in their heads (a bit like sitting in the U.N. general assembly with translator headphones on). They may then repeat back to the teen the "translation" of these statements, which is "I know you don't like what we're doing, but it *is* what we're going to do." Parents may need considerable support from their therapist to remain firm and consistent in the face of "emotional blackmail."

## Homework

Implement all written behavioral contracts, or continue to implement the point system. Parents should be encouraged to call for assistance if needed over the coming week. Ask parents to get a progress report from the teen's guidance counselor or teachers for discussion at Session 9. They should also gather copies of relevant school materials such as recent report cards, warning notices, school-based testing reports, and most importantly any written educational plans.

# Grounding

## Goal

- To train parents in the use of an effective grounding method as punishment for selected teen misbehavior.

## Materials Required

- Parent Handout for Step 8
    Grounding

## Session Outline

- Review of parent management tactics to date.
- Discuss use of grounding for more serious problems.

## Homework

- Explain grounding procedure to teen.
- Use grounding if necessary.

Have parents describe their use of the behavioral contracts or the point system, with a focus on how comfortable they are with the mechanics of the procedures and how consistent they are in awarding privileges or points and following through with penalties. Be sure to commend parents for practicing these strategies. Refine their implementation as needed. If parents did not do their homework, get them to clarify the nature of the impasse and problem-solve so they may be able to proceed over the coming week.

# Grounding

Give the rationale for using grounding: Penalties must fit the crime. Taking away points or privileges can be very effective for not completing daily chores or for violations of most household rules, but may not be enough for more serious behavioral problems. Grounding may be used for more difficult problem behaviors. Grounding, like "time out" for younger children, formally means "time out from reinforcement." Therefore, it involves withholding all forms of positive activity as punishment.

Explain how parents tend to misuse or overuse grounding, such as the following examples:

- "You're grounded for a week"—until the parent cools off and remembers some important event the teen is scheduled for, lets him/her go, and undermines his/her authority.
- "You're grounded"—meaning the teen stays in the house but watches TV, uses the phone, and so forth. This is not "time out from reinforcement." (*We* would personally love to be grounded for as long as possible if that's what it's like.)
- "You're grounded for a week"—after a brief time, the ADHD teen no longer connects the punishment with whatever it was he/she did. Instead, he/she feels resentful, and the grounding does not even effectively alter his/her behavior.
- "You're grounded for a week"—then a couple of days later the teen does something else, so, "You're grounded for another week," and so on and so forth. The teen may end up being grounded all winter!
- "You're grounded"—but the parents cannot be there to monitor what the teen is doing, so he/she violates the restriction in the parents' absence, thus undermining parental authority.

Give parents the handout on grounding and have them read it before proceeding with a description of the procedure.

Effective grounding of defiant teens should be short and to the point. Essentially, grounding means "house arrest": for a few hours to 2 days maximum, the teen has no access to anything the parent would define as a privilege, and might have to perform some sort of "work detail" (such as sweeping out the garage, washing windows, etc., for no pay). The teen should be informed ahead of time what sort of behavior will lead to grounding, or told that you will issue a warning when he/she is in danger of being grounded (e.g., if the teen is having some sort of tantrum, the parent could start by removing a privilege, then give one warning, and follow up with grounding). The parent must be able to be at home to monitor the grounding, so it might have to be somewhat delayed. The teen can be grounded for the rest of the day, for a full day, or for the weekend. Once grounding is over, the parent reminds the teen of the behaviors that will lead to grounding in the future, but then goes on with the daily routine in a business-like fashion. Parents need the plan, too, so they don't react out of anger. When very angry, many parents use grounding as a form of retaliation or revenge, rather than discipline or education.

## Common Family Reactions

Some parents express confusion over the meaning of the term "time out." Parents need to be aware that there are two different definitions of "time out." As noted above, "time out" may be a punishment procedure used with children under the age of approximately 10 years that is similar in nature to grounding, which is "time out from reinforcement." However, "time out" can also be thought of as a coping strategy for adults and teenagers when they become so angry or emotionally aroused that they cannot control their behavior or their words. In this respect, "time out" is similar to "count to ten": the person removes him/herself from the confrontation in order to "cool off." "Time out" as a coping strategy is extremely beneficial to families with defiant teenagers, once they learn to use it effectively, and may turn out to be an important coping strategy for the teen to use in other relationships. When used this way, "time out" is not a punishment. It is a constructive response to emotional volatility. Parents may suggest that the teen take a "time out" if his/her anger is clearly escalating, and warn the teen that if not he/she may face either a penalty or grounding.

## Homework

Choose one or two behaviors for which grounding is to be used. Have parents keep a diary over the coming week of any use of either grounding or "time out." Even more than before, urge parents to call for assistance as needed, because grounding can be one of the hardest procedures to implement correctly. Parents of older teens (age 17 or 18) may not be advised to utilize grounding, either because the teen has the ability simply to walk out of the house (perhaps even drive away in his/her own car) or developmentally is too mature to respond constructively to this strategy. In these cases, parents must construct a hierarchy of penalties (i.e., privileges that are in the parents' control to take away, from least meaningful to most meaningful) that they will utilize in response to a similar hierarchy of negative behaviors (from least severe to most severe).

# School Advocacy

## *Goals*

1. To review with parents the nature of any behavior or academic problems the teen may be demonstrating at school.
2. To review the accommodations schools can make for students with developmental disabilities or special needs.

## *Materials Required*

- Parent Handouts for Step 9

   Accommodations for Improving Teen School Performance
   1991 Memorandum from the U.S. Department of Education

- Issues Checklist

## *Session Outline*

- Review and refine implementation of the grounding procedure.
- Review and refine other major aspects of the program to date.
- Discuss concerns related to the teen's school performance.
- Inform parents about where ADHD is covered by law (e.g., the Individuals with Disabilities in Education Act and the Americans with Disabilities Act).

## *Homework*

- Consult with school personnel if necessary.
- Continue previously taught methods.

Discuss with parents all efforts to use grounding this past week. Review the diary they kept for any problems with inappropriate or excessive use of grounding, excessively long groundings, or any parental reluctance to use grounding. Also discuss the teen's reaction to grounding, especially coercion or escalation in hostility. Once again, discuss the possibility that parents may have to call outside authorities such as the police or juvenile court if they feel that the teen's or their own safety is in danger.

Review implementation of the entire program to date. Diagram for parents the components of the program, emphasizing the balance of positive and negative strategies, as well as the absence of physical coercion or yelling (in this program, punishments are things we *take away*, not things we *inflict upon*):

| *Positive* | *Negative* |
|---|---|
| Nonjudgmental positive time | Ignoring minor misbehavior |
| Praise | Giving penalties |
| Incentives/privileges | Grounding |

Be sure to commend any success to date. Refine program implementation as needed. If parents are not using any aspect of the program on a regular basis, get them to clarify what is getting in the way and problem-solve so they may continue.

## Review of School-Based Concerns

Give parents the handout on classroom accommodations for improving teen school performance. Describe "reasonable accommodations" in a middle school or high school setting, with examples such as the following:

- The guidance counselor acts as the "coach" in school, checking in with teachers weekly to monitor progress, meeting with teen briefly each morning to review the day's schedule and assist with organization and time management.
- The ADHD teen does as much homework as possible in school, preferably in a monitored study hall or a resource room study hall.
- The ADHD teen is allowed two sets of text books, the teacher's phone number or e-mail address to contact about assignments, a peer tutor or study buddy to assist with recording of assignments, photocopies of the class syllabus or lecture outlines.
- The ADHD teen is allowed access to technological supports, such as tape recorders for class lectures, calculators, laptop computers for notetaking in class, word processor for written assignments, or computerized instructional programs.
- Classroom teachers utilize multimethod instructional strategies, such as an overhead projector with lecture outlines or assignments on it; cooperative group learning; art, music, dance, or drama; hands-on projects; computer products; and props of any sort to stimulate and entertain as well as teach.

- Classroom teachers utilize multimethod assessment procedures, such as allowing the student to give oral responses to test questions, to dictate responses that someone else transcribes, to take an untimed test, or to take a test in a separate classroom with fewer distractions and with an adult to make sure he/she doesn't rush through it.

## Homework

If there are problems pertaining to completion of a reasonable amount of homework at home, review with parents the context and timing surrounding homework. Does the teenager record his homework in an assignment book? Are parents nagging too much about homework? Does the teen have someone to call if he has questions about homework? Have specific limits on the time to complete homework been established? Is the setting for doing homework appropriate? Does the teenager have an organized approach to doing homework? Do the parents monitor completion of homework?

Have parents stipulate a time for homework to be done each day. The teen will then be rewarded with access to a privilege or points if homework is completed, or a penalty will be imposed if homework is not completed. In addressing homework problems, however, it is critical for parents to be confident that the amount of work the teachers are assigning is reasonable for a student with ADHD.

The therapist might develop a comprehensive behavioral contract to enhance completion of homework. The following example of such a contract for Michael Adams, an adolescent with ADHD, has proven clinically useful (Robin, 1998):

### A Homework Contract for Michael Adams

I, Michael Adams, together with my parents, teachers, guidance counselor, and principal, agree to carry out to the best of our ability the following homework plan:

I. **Keeping Track of Assignments**
   A. My teachers will write the assignments on the board every day. They will also give a copy of all the assignments for the week to Mrs. Smith, my guidance counselor, each Monday. She will keep a copy and mail a copy home to my parents.

   B. I will write down the assignment from the board every day before I leave each class. I will write it on the back of the section divider for the section of my looseleaf binder for each class. I will read over what I have written down to make sure I understand it. I will ask the teacher to explain any assignment I do not understand.

   C. During my last period study hall, I will read over each assignment that I have written down and make sure I understand what I am being asked to do. I will make a list of all of the materials I need to bring home and gather them from my locker. My study hall teacher agrees to give me a hall pass during last period to go to my locker and find any materials I need.

## II. Bringing Home Materials

A. I will bring home all of the materials I have gathered as well as the binder in which I have written my assignments down.

B. My mother agrees to ask me nicely one time without nagging to see my list of assignments. I agree to show it to her without a big hassle or an attitude.

C. As a backup in case I forget to write the assignment down, I will pick a study buddy in each of my classes, get that person's phone number, and post those phone numbers on the refrigerator door.

## III. Schedule and Setting for Doing Homework

A. From Sunday through Thursday, I agree to work on homework from 6:00 P.M. to 8:00 P.M. If I finish early, I will show my completed work to a parent, and if he/she agrees that it is completed, I can do whatever I want.

B. I will do my homework at the big desk in the den. I can listen to soft music with headphones, but no loud rock. If I find myself getting distracted, I will take a short break, do something physical (not using the telephone), and start working again.

C. My mother will remind me once without nagging to start on my homework at 6:00 P.M. I will start without an attitude.

## IV. Daily Plan for Organizing Homework Completion

A. With help from my mother, I will make an organized plan for each night's homework. This plan will guide me in which subject I will do first, second, etc. It will also divide up homework time between assignments due tomorrow and long-term assignments. My mother agrees to permit me to determine the order of doing homework.

B. My plan will estimate the time needed to complete each assignment, as well as how I will check each assignment for accuracy, completeness, and legibility.

C. The plan will specify how often I will take breaks during homework time, how long the breaks will be, and how large assignments will be divided into smaller units.

D. The plan will specify where I will put the completed assignments and how I will make sure I turn the work in.

## V. Medication. I agree to take a dose of Ritalin at 5:00 P.M., Sunday through Thursday, to help me concentrate on homework.

## VI. Turning in Assignments

A. As I finish an assignment, I will put it in the section of my binder for that class.

B. I will do my best to remember to hand in each assignment.

## VII. Feedback. My teachers agree to tell me how I did within 2 days after I hand in an assignment. They also agree to send my parents feedback on how many of the last week's assign-

ments were turned in on time, when they send the next week's assignment list. The guidance counselor will collect these materials from the teachers and mail them out.

VIII. **Rewards.** My parents agree to let me make 20 minutes of long-distance phone calls to my girlfriend each night that I do my homework. If I do my homework for five nights in a row, they agree to let me make 45 minutes of long-distance phone calls on the weekend.

| Signed, | Michael Adams | Robert Adams | Barbara Adams |
| --- | --- | --- | --- |
| | Bill Jones, Principal | Brenda Smith, Guidance Counselor | |
| | Millie Broadbent, Algebra | Tom Jones, English | |
| | Darla Breeze, French | William Sonoma, Chemistry | |
| | F.A.O. Schwartz, Gym | Neiman Marcus, History | |

(Robin, 1998, pp. 274–275)

## Educational Rights

Discuss the educational rights of children diagnosed with ADHD as outlined in the handout "1991 Memorandum from the U.S. Department of Education. The public school student with a disability that impairs his academic functioning is entitled to services via any one or a combination of three possible mechanisms:

1. An individualized educational plan (IEP) written and implemented by the special education department that addresses both a diagnosed specific learning disability as well as ADHD.
2. An IEP written and implemented by the special education department that addresses only ADHD, which is defined under special education law as a "health impairment."
3. A Section 504 Plan written by the school's coordinator for the Americans with Disabilities Act, to be followed by all regular education teachers working with the child.

Highlight the importance of teachers needing to have proper knowledge and understanding of ADHD as well as administrative support; otherwise, they very likely will not be receptive to incorporating any recommended accommodations. Encourage parents to take an active role in their teen's schooling and work closely and in collaboration with teachers and the guidance counselor. They may also want to investigate local parent support groups or parent advisory committees for specific advice regarding their own school system.

## Conclusion for Steps 1–9

Discuss how to address behavior problems by "playing detective" and hypothesizing what the nature of the problem might be. In constructing a theory, parents can run through each step of the program, including the nature of ADHD, the four-factor model of teen misbehavior, and the situational consequences for the behavior problem. They should be particularly on the lookout for any lack of consistency in their parenting style.

## Common Family Reactions

Many families have experienced considerable frustration with the public school system. It is important for the therapist to be aware that there are always two sides to such a story. Most schools are overwhelmed by budgetary demands, as well as the demands of increasingly larger classrooms, with many students who have individual needs. The "inclusion" model of education may place enormous pressures on regular classroom teachers. This does not excuse discrimination against a student with ADHD, but the therapist needs to exercise diplomacy in dealing with angry parents, advising that, as in this program, a business-like approach should be used to address any controversies.

## Additional Interventions for School-Based Problems

A comprehensive analysis of the educational problems of adolescents who are defiant and/ or have ADHD goes beyond the scope of this manual, which focuses primarily on home-based problems. However, many of the adolescents participating in this family treatment program will also benefit from such interventions. Readers interested in procedures for addressing additional school-related concerns might consult Markel and Greenbaum (1996) or Robin (1998).

## Homework

Parents should consult with school personnel regarding any proposed changes to the teen's education plan. Address academic homework problems as necessary.

Inform the teen that he will be attending the remaining nine therapy sessions with his parents. Both parents and teen complete the Issues Checklist (found in Part III) before the next session.

# Introduction to Problem-Solving Communication Training

## *Comment on Sequencing*

In our clinical use of this defiant teen program, the second part of the program (Steps 10–18) was presented in the order shown here. However, clinical experience has suggested that several changes in the sequencing of these steps may at times be useful. First, some families benefit from having Step 15, on beliefs and expectations, presented after Step 10. In Step 15, families develop realistic expectations and appropriate attributions. Unrealistic expectations and distorted beliefs may interfere with learning and applying problem-solving communication skills (PSCT) for some families. Second, in some families, extremely negative communication side-tracks them from problem solving, and they can never get through an entire problem-solving discussion without a major argument. Such families need communication training before problem-solving training. In such cases, it is best to insert Step 13 after Step 10.

## *Goals*

1. To introduce the principles of PSCT.
2. To engage the teen in the therapy endeavor.
3. To encourage cautious optimism and some enthusiasm in both the teen and the parents about PSCT.
4. To familiarize the family with the problem-solving model and coach the family in practicing these steps with a contrived/mock issue.

*Materials Required*

- Parent Handouts for Step 10

    Steps to Better Problem Solving
    Problem-Solving Worksheet
    Problem-Solving Exercise

- Videotape for teens on ADHD

*Session Outline*

- Meet individually with the parents: Introduce the principles of PSCT.
- Meet individually with the teen to establish rapport and review his/her questions about ADHD or the family therapy.
- Meet with the family and introduce the rationale behind PSCT methods.
- Construct a hierarchy of parent–teen conflicts from mildest to hottest using the Issues Checklist results.
- Introduce the steps to problem solving, using instructions, modeling, behavior rehearsal, and feedback.

*Homework*

- Each family member separately completes the Problem-Solving Exercise.

# Principles of PSCT

Explain to parents that now that they have learned how to apply the principles of parent management to their adolescent, it is time to involve their adolescent in the treatment session and directly work on resolving conflicts and communicating with their adolescent. This session will prepare the parents for learning new methods of interacting with their adolescent by introducing the principles underlying problem solving and communication, and then teaching parents to apply these principles to the resolution of conflicts with their adolescent. Introduce and discuss each of the following principles (see Chapter 3 of Part I for more details):

- Gradually grant increasing independence.
- Distinguish negotiable from nonnegotiable issues.
- Involve adolescents in problem solving negotiable issues.
- Maintain good communication.
- Develop reasonable expectations.

## Individual Meeting with the Adolescent

Next, meet with the adolescent for no more than 10–15 minutes to reestablish rapport and prepare for the family session. Remember that you have not seen the adolescent since the initial assessment, and you have been instructing the parents to apply principles of behavior management to the adolescent. The adolescent may perceive you as someone who is telling the parents how to control him/her, so if you expect the adolescent to cooperate in the forthcoming family sessions, you need to reestablish your relationship with him/her. Start with a minute or two of social "chit chat" designed to draw the teen into the session. Comment positively about some aspect of the teen's appearance, if appropriate, or ask about some recent activity of the teen. Next, briefly explain that now that you have completed the process of teaching the teen's parents basic principles of behavior management, it is time to involve the teen in learning how to resolve conflicts with the parents. Ask if the teen has any comments or reactions to the interventions that the parents have already been implementing.

When appropriate, ask if the teen has any questions about ADHD. You may wish to show a short video such as *ADHD in Adolescence: Our Point of View* (Schubiner, 1995), which depicts five teenagers discussing their experiences with ADHD. Describe how the combination of normal adolescent development ADHD and may lead to increased verbal conflicts between parents and the teen, which will be the focus of the next nine sessions. Readers interested in more information about how to educate adolescents to accept ADHD should consult Robin (1998).

Use this time to encourage teen involvement in treatment. Stress that the teen very likely wants things from the parents, but to get them, he/she will need to learn better methods of negotiating for them. Emphasize that negotiation may mean giving in on some things to get other things that the teen wants. The teen's views and requests should be supported as much as possible in these sessions, provided that what the teen seeks is reasonable. Stress that treatment cannot succeed without the teen's cooperation.

Note that occasionally during the later sessions that the teen attends with the parents, you may decide to spend a short additional time alone with the teen. Sometimes, teens perceive family therapists as siding with their parents. During another individual meeting, the purpose would primarily be to reestablish rapport with the teen so that he/she can maintain enthusiasm for the program. This should not happen routinely, and the teen should be encouraged to bring any specific frustrations back to the sessions with his parents.

## Family Session

Meet with the parents and teen together. Explain that parent–teen conflict is mostly *verbal* arguments about specific issues. These sessions will focus on changing the way family members talk to each other when in conflict—especially conflict that escalates in frequency and intensity. Possibly use the "acting school" metaphor: First we will learn a "script," that is, the specific problem-solving steps that will be utilized for each and every issue addressed in these sessions. Then we will work on "delivery," that is, *how* family members communicate with each other. Finally, we will focus on "motivation," that is, the unrealistic or irrational beliefs that family members sometimes hold about each other and that fuel angry feelings.

## The Issues Checklist

Create a list of topics for discussion from the Issues Checklist (found in Part III) previously completed by parents and teens (list these topics in order of severity from "5" down to "1"). In these sessions, you will work from the mildest to the most severe (take note of any differences in priorities between teen and parents on any topic). Note next to each issue whether it came from the parent, adolescent, or both Issues Checklists. For example, here is a list from one of our clinic cases:

Intensity 5: Most angry
Fighting with brothers and sisters (parent)
Talking back to parents (parent)
Who should be friends (teen)
Coming home on time (parent)
Getting to school on time (parent)
Intensity 4: Somewhat less angry
Homework (teen, parent)
Getting low grades in school (parent)
Getting in trouble in school (teen, parent)
Cleaning up bedroom (parent)
Lying (parent, teen)
Intensity 3: A little angry
Cursing (teen, parent)
Helping out around the house (parent)
Smoking (teen)
Getting up in the morning (parent)
Intensity 2: Mildly angry
Playing the stereo too loudly (teen)
Messing up the house (parent)
Bothering parents when they want to be left alone (parent)
How money is spent (teen)
Intensity 1: Mild
Turning off lights (teen)
Putting feet on the furniture (parent, teen)
Using the TV (parent, teen)
Cleanliness (parent)
Which clothes to wear (parent, teen)

## Give the Rationale for Problem Solving

Introduce the problem-solving steps, displaying a chart with the steps (the first handout) that can be visually referred to during the session. Talk about how this model has been used in the business world to save companies on the verge of bankruptcy and in international diplomacy, such as between Israel and Palestine. Explain the distinction between nonnegotiable and negotiable issues and explain that problem solving is used to resolve the negotiable issues. For example, use of drugs and violence are not negotiable, but cleaning up the bedroom and how money is spent are negotiable. Explain that problem solving is a way for adolescents to be involved in making decisions regarding issues that affect them, and that everyone gets to give their opinions, resulting in a compromise solution being reached.

## Introduce Each Step of Problem Solving

It works best to introduce one step of problem solving at a time, and walk the family through that step with a hypothetical problem. This maintains involvement by requiring frequent interaction. Display a chart with the problem-solving steps and have one family member fill in a copy of the Problem-Solving Worksheet (the second handout) while you are doing this. Use an example such as the following:

I know a boy named Billy who is about to turn 16. Billy wants to have a birthday party and invite 100 of his closest friends, and he doesn't want his parents home for the party. His parents aren't happy about the idea.

*Define the problem.* Give the following rationale: "Step one is to define the problem. The problem is defined by making a short, nonaccusing statement of what the other person is doing, what the situation is, and why it is a problem. Each person has a turn to define the problem. Speak in terms of 'I' rather than 'you' to avoid blaming others. Different family members will have different perspectives on the problem, and this is perfectly acceptable. Family members do not have to agree on each other's problem definitions. Billy might say, 'Mom and Dad, I get embarrassed when you are around during a teenager party so I don't want you to be there.' Saying this is much better than saying that his parents are a couple of old 'fuddy duddies' for not realizing that everyone has parties like this. The first statement is not a putdown, and in it he is taking responsibility for his own feelings. Billy's mother might say, 'I don't want you to have a party without an adult present because I am worried that your friends may make poor choices and get themselves or you in trouble, or mess up the house.'" Ask the family members to give definitions of the birthday party problem from their perspectives, and give them feedback about their statements.

After each person defines the problem, another family member will be asked to repeat the definition back to the speaker, to check for accuracy of understanding. The speaker will be asked either to acknowledge that the listener correctly understood the definition or to correct any misunderstandings. Illustrate how the problem definition statements regarding Billy's party might be paraphrased back and verified for understanding, and ask the family members to try paraphrasing and verifying them.

After each person has practiced defining the problem and paraphrasing another's definition, point out how there are several different points of view of the problem, and that this is natural under the circumstances.

\* \* \*

*Generate the solutions.* Provide the following rationale: "Now that you have defined the problem, you need to think of some solutions. You will take turns listing ideas until we have at least 12 possible solutions to the problem. This is the time to be creative, without being concerned that other family members are going to be critical. Suggest anything that comes to mind, even if it seems silly. Don't judge the ideas, though; that comes later. Remember, you don't have to do it just because you said it. This is called brainstorming. One person will write down the ideas on the worksheet for later reference." The therapist will need to police the restriction against premature evaluations vigorously. Although we have suggested that the therapist ask the family to generate at least 12 solutions, it should be noted that the therapist needs to watch to see that the solutions being generated go beyond the family members' initial positions and are possible bases for compromise. Usually, 12 solutions are sufficient for this to happen.

Guide the family to generate 12 solutions to Billy's birthday party solution, taking turns. If they run out of ideas early, suggest a number of outlandish ideas in a humorous fashion. For example, you might suggest, "Parents spy on the party through closed circuit video cameras set up in every room and relayed by satellite to another location."

\* \* \*

*Evaluate the solutions.* Then, in step 3, each family member (including the teen) has a chance to evaluate each solution, giving it a "+" or a "−", based on whether or not they like the solution or whether or not they think it is realistic. These ratings are recorded next to the solution in the appropriate column of the worksheet. An evaluation statement projects whether the idea will solve the speaker's definition of the problem and also includes an evaluative rating of "+" or "−". Sometimes family members omit the discussion of whether the idea will work; the therapist should prompt them to include such a statement because this helps teach means–ends or consequential thinking skills. The therapist should illustrate evaluative statements and ask the family to evaluate their list of 12 solutions for Billy's birthday party problem, recording their evaluations on the worksheet.

\* \* \*

*Select the option most agreeable to all.* After each solution has been evaluated, explain to the family that their goal is to reach a decision that everyone can live with and with which everyone will have to give up something to get something. This is the essence of negotiation. Ask the secretary to read aloud the ideas rated "+" by everyone. If one or more ideas were rated positively by all, congratulate the family on reaching an agreement and ask them to combine these ideas into an overall solution. If no ideas were rated positively by all, help them negotiate a compromise.

Ask the family to review their evaluations of Billy's birthday party solution and to reach an agreement on an idea that they all rated positively. In cases where no compromise was reached, look for an idea on which they came close to agreement. Clearly state the gap between the various positions. Ask the family to bridge the gap between their various positions by suggesting additional ideas in-between their respective positions. Have them evaluate these additional ideas and try to reach an agreement. Robin and Foster (1989) have outlined other approaches to resolving such impasses.

\* \* \*

*Plan to implement the solution.* Explain to the family that the goal of implementation planning is for the family to specify the details so that the agreed-upon solution can be put into operation. These details include (1) who will do what, when, and where; (2) who will monitor compliance with the agreement, and how monitoring will be carried out (with charts or verbally); (3) the consequences for compliance or noncompliance with the agreement; (4) what, if any, performance reminders will be given; (5) exactly what constitutes compliance (e.g., how clean must the adolescent's room be); and (6) what difficulties are anticipated in carrying out the agreement. In essence, a behavioral contract may be written regarding compliance with the agreed-upon solution.

These steps are essential in the case of ADHD teens, since we know that they need performance prompts and immediate consequences to maintain behavior. The therapist should review the implementation section of the Problem-Solving Worksheet with the family. This section guides them in fleshing out the necessary details for a successful implementation of the solution. The family should complete an implementation plan for the hypothetical birthday party problem. Explain to the family that the next step involves actually going home and implementing the agreed-upon solution.

\* \* \*

*Evaluate the implementation of the solution.* Explain that after a week or two of trying the solution out at home, the family can then determine whether or not the solution is working. If it is not, they may need to go back to the worksheet to find another solution, or possibly even redefine the problem. In some cases, the solution is a good one but one member of the family is not motivated to stick with it consistently. In this case, adding a negative consequence for not using the solution may be a good idea. Remember that a consequence (positive or negative) might actually be a solution that a family member proposes. For example, the problem might be "coming home on time" and a proposed solution might be "If you are late, you will not go out with your friends on the following day." Ask the family to imagine that they implemented a solution to the birthday party problem and to anticipate some difficulties that might come up during the implementation. Ask them to speculate how they could deal with these problems.

## Common Family Reactions

Families will often draw a blank after generating three or four possible solutions. It is fine for the therapist to contribute one or two in order to teach family members how to be more creative. As these sessions progress, you may want occasionally to suggest a "provocative" solution that will generate a productive discussion during the evaluation step. For example, you might suggest "Billy could quit school," "Billy could move out," or "Billy's parents could let him do whatever he wants."

It is also possible that you will not complete all of the activities scheduled in Step 10 during a single session. as it contains a very full agenda. If you do not complete all of these activities, continue them during Step 11, which does not have as tightly packed an agenda.

## Homework

Send the family home with the Problem-Solving Exercise (the third handout), which they are to work on separately and bring with them for the next session.

# Practicing Problem Solving

## Goals

1. To begin to get the family used to the problem-solving routine.
2. To work through a low-intensity problem.
3. To complete any activities left over from Step 10.

## Materials Required

- Blank Problem-Solving Worksheet for homework (have a chart with the problem-solving steps displayed for each session from now on)

## Session Outline

- Review the Problem-Solving Exercise.
- Select a low-intensity problem from the list generated last time to work through in this session.

## Homework

- Implement any solutions generated from the session's discussion.
- Practice and tape record a problem-solving discussion at home.

Review the homework, highlighting the *objective*, *nonjudgmental* aspect of problem definition. Highlight any obvious similarities between the responses of the teenager and the responses of the parents: Parents are often surprised to see that their child has a similar reaction to the hypothetical situations. Be very encouraging and enthusiastic about their attempts to generate possible solutions to the long-distance telephone problem from their homework exercise. Keep the discussion impersonal at this point, emphasizing the mechanics of the problem-solving "script," while avoiding getting into personal issues.

## Practice Problem Solving

Select a low-priority or low-intensity problem from the family's responses to the Issues Checklist (but not an issue that the family tells you is no longer meaningful to them). Indicate that you will balance your selection of topics generated by the parents and the adolescent. If you select a topic generated by the parent in this session, be sure to select one generated by the adolescent in the next session. Move through as many steps as possible. Coach the family to follow the outline of problem-solving steps, and focus your efforts on intensive skill building. Correct faulty problem definitions, stop premature evaluations, and prompt complete evaluations. Give as much feedback as necessary to shape improved responses. This session and the next provide the opportunity to refine the family members' ability to apply the components of problem solving. Be as directive as necessary in guiding them toward reaching a solution that they can implement at home. Spend an adequate amount of time coaching the family to plan the details necessary for a successful implementation of the solution, and have them record those details in the appropriate sections of the worksheet. With more skilled families, you may be able to get through all the steps and select a solution that will then be implemented over the coming week. Families who did not complete the discussion in the session should complete it as part of their homework. Families should take the worksheets with them either to post in a prominent spot at home or to keep in a folder for easy reference.

Pay particular attention to the possible need to tailor elements of the model to the needs of an ADHD adolescent, who may experience difficulty sitting through an entire problem-solving discussion. Recognize when the adolescent's yawning, fidgety, whining behavior represents the mental fatigue and burnout common with ADHD adolescents rather than truly oppositional behavior, and do not let the parents overreact inappropriately. Keep your comments and the parents' comments brief and to the point, talk in an animated and humorous style, and frequently bring the adolescent into the discussion. Gauge the amount of time that the adolescent can "last" and consider having shorter sessions or taking a short "stretch break" in the middle of the session to permit movement. Simplify the steps of problem solving, for example, by having the parents brainstorm and evaluate the solutions, then presenting the adolescent with two or three choices to consider. Finally, when appropriate, time the therapy session so that the adolescent's stimulant medication is in effect during the session.

## Common Family Reactions

Someone does not do his/her homework. Don't dwell on it; simply have that person generate answers during the discussion. Especially if it is the teen, don't "ally" yourself against any one family member. Emphasize the need to work together on homework discussions for the remainder of the sessions.

## Homework

Complete the problem-solving discussion, if not already completed in the session. Implement the solution generated from the day's discussion.

Ask the family to use a tape recorder for discussions at home (or loan them one, although you may want to get a deposit against its return). Make sure that if one parent isn't able to come to sessions regularly, they participate as much as possible in taped discussions at home. Assign a low-intensity problem off the family's list for a taped discussion at home. Families should discuss for at least 15 minutes, but stop if the discussion becomes too heated and angry. They should use a blank Problem-Solving Worksheet and go through the same steps that were used in this session, keeping the handout on Steps to Better Problem Solving in front of them during the discussion. As in the sessions, one family member volunteers to be the "scribe" and record the entries onto the sheet. This responsibility should rotate among the parents and teen.

# Practicing Problem Solving, Continued

### Goals

1. To review solution implementation and problem-solving discussion.
2. To work through another, slightly higher intensity, problem off the family's list.

### Materials Required

- Blank Problem-Solving Worksheet for discussion of homework

### Session Outline

- Review the homework exercise.
- Continue to practice the steps to better problem solving.

### Homework

- Implement any agreed-upon solutions.
- Practice and tape a problem-solving discussion at home.

Collect the tape of the home problem-solving discussion from the family. (Review it before their next session; note not only breakdowns in the flow of the problem-solving steps but also errors in communication style, and focus on them in the next session.) Discuss how the family felt about holding a discussion at home with the tape recorder, and how successful they were at generating solutions. If they did not do the homework, make *that* the topic of a problem-solving discussion in this session.

Review the implementation of the solution generated in the last session. Did the family successfully implement the solution? Get an independent report from each family member. If they successfully implemented the solution, how well is it working? Are any modifications necessary? Praise them for successful implementations and instruct them to continue with the solution. If the solution was not successfully implemented, investigate what went wrong, objectively but persistently. Did the family try to implement the solution? If not, why not? If they tried but did not succeed, was there resistance to the solution from one or more family members? Who was resistant, and what type of resistance was it? Did negative communication sidetrack them? Was there general mistrust and hostility? Did ADHD-related factors such as forgetfulness and disorganization interfere with the implementation of the solution? Did a family crisis occur and eclipse the importance of dealing with this solution?

Using the answers to these questions, guide the family in modifying the solution so that they can have more success implementing it. Place their negative outcome within a problem-solving framework—that is, indicate that something went wrong at one of the stages of problem solving, impeding them from coming up with the optimal solution or implementation plan—rather than letting them think that certain family members failed or were irresponsible. Help them figure out what went wrong and plan to overcome it. If necessary, make this the topic of today's problem-solving discussion rather than a new topic. Incorporate another try at implementation into the homework for this session.

## Conduct Another Problem-Solving Discussion

Select a moderately low-intensity problem from the Issues Checklist for the formal problem-solving discussion. If space in your office permits, you may choose at this point to rearrange the furniture so that the family members are seated in a circle facing each other and you are sitting outside and behind the circle. This arrangement encourages the family to problem-solve with each other and to leave you out of the discussion. You will still provide some commentary from outside the circle, but try to keep it to a minimum during their discussion. You can take notes of their communication-style errors for the next session; wait until the discussion is finished or until they become stuck before giving corrective feedback. Continue, as in the last session, to target and correct faulty problem-solving statements, refining the family members' skills.

## Common Family Reactions

Sometimes one family member will take on most of the responsibility to generate possible solutions. If this happens, instruct family members to take turns suggesting a solution. If, for example, only the mother is suggesting solutions, then it is unlikely that the teen is going to end up giving a positive evaluation to any of the proposed solutions. It is acceptable for the therapist to be somewhat directive and require that each family member contribute some solutions, even if those solutions seem unrealistic.

## Homework

Implement any solutions generated from today's session. Continue implementation of the solution from the last session. Select a problem for discussion at home with the tape recorder.

# Introduction to Communication Skills

## *Goals*

1. To continue developing family's expertise in problem solving.
2. To introduce communication skills.
3. To teach general principles of good communication.
4. To identify and begin to correct specific negative communication styles.

## *Materials Required*

- Parent Handout for Step 13

    Communication Habits (display this chart in your office during each session from now on)

    Blank Problem-Solving Worksheet for homework

## *Session Outline*

- Review homework assignment on problem solving.
- Give advice for improvements as needed.
- Request tape of home problem-solving discussion from the family (review it before their next session; note not only breakdowns in the flow of the problem-solving steps but also communication-style errors to focus on in the next session).

## *Homework*

- Practice using improved communication habits.
- Conduct another problem-solving discussion.

Review the implementation of previous solutions. Do they need to be modified? Does the family need to revisit a problem discussion to come up with a new solution? If so, then you should have that discussion now.

## Communication Skills

Introduce the following three general principles of good communication:

1. Listen when your teen/parent is in the mood to talk, but don't force him/her to open up.
2. Use active listening to encourage your teen/parent to express opinions and feelings.
3. Honestly express how you feel, good or bad, without being hurtful to your listeners.

Explain the rationale for these principles. Adolescents may go for days or weeks without having the urge to open up to their parents, but then for no apparent reason, they suddenly need to talk, often at inconvenient times for parents. Parents need to make themselves available at such times. Define and model active listening, and ask the parents and the adolescent to practice it for a few moments, perhaps using the practice topic of describing how their day has been going. Active listening occurs when the listener does not simply hear what the speaker is saying but attempts to mentally summarize the gist or point of the commentary. This can be taught by having the listener paraphrase or summarize what the speaker has just said. Discuss the importance of the listener expressing feelings and opinions, including anger, frustration, sadness, and other negative emotions, but point out that such expressions can be made without demeaning the other person. Ask the family to start applying these principles to all of their communications with each other.

Now turn your attention to specific negative communication styles, using your chart of negative styles and their alternatives. Explain each of the negative habits in some detail. Ask family members to give recent examples of the negative communication habits in action in their family. As they give each example of a negative habit, guide them to examine alternative, more positive replacement behaviors such as those listed on the right-hand side of the handout. Emphasize that people usually use the bad habits when they are angry, so it is important to use "Count to 10, or take a hike" as a coping strategy to cool off before having a discussion. Each family member should begin to monitor him/herself for these habits, substituting the positive alternatives whenever possible. Also, as family members begin to monitor themselves on these habits, they should *not* monitor each other—this can just provoke more conflict.

Based on this review of negative communication habits, select a few key communication targets to address directly in each family. Explain to the family that you will stop their interactions as needed when you hear and see the negative habits occurring, and you will ask them to "replay the scene" engaging in a more positive communication behavior. We call this systematic communication training. Have the family begin a new problem-solving discussion, this time on a more heated topic, possibly related to school performance. Interrupt as needed to identify communication-style errors, and suggest positive alternatives. Also, catch problem-solving errors. Arrange the chairs so that you are outside the discussion, if desired. Do not expect to finish the entire problem-solving discussion during the session; concentrate primarily on correcting negative communication. The family can finish the discussion at home, if necessary.

## Common Family Reactions

*ADHD communication.* In families with ADHD adolescents, the parents may report that their teens do many things that could be considered examples of negative communication. If the parent were to attempt to correct every one of these behaviors, it would tax the patience of even the most reflective and tolerant adult. These negative communication behaviors just happen, often without premeditation or even awareness on the part of the adolescent; that is the biological legacy of ADHD. Giving feedback on all such behaviors might also damage the adolescent's self-esteem, because of the continuous stream of negative feedback that would be necessary. In such situations, the therapist must teach parents how to prioritize which communication targets to correct and which to ignore, that is, pick their battles wisely. We find it useful to teach parents to distinguish between *truly negative* and *truly ADHD* communication. Truly negative communication is intentional, premeditated proactive, critical, and demeaning, aimed at the weaknesses of the other person, or designed to hurt the other person or manipulate him/her into doing what the speaker wants. Truly ADHD communication is also negative and hurtful, but it is reactive, spontaneous, impulsive, nonsensical, and stupidly executed, in a manner that is unlikely to get the other person to do what the speaker wants; it occurs under conditions of fatigue, external stress, or threat, when external circumstances further erode the ADHD individual's already impaired inhibitory control. Family members need to give a high priority to targeting the truly negative communication, and basically ignore the truly ADHD communication. Only after all of the truly negative communication has been corrected and no longer occurs should a parent devote time and effort to the ADHD communication.

*Insufficient information.* There will be times when a family member will generate a possible solution that cannot be effectively evaluated because not enough information is available to pass judgment. For example, the family of one young man was addressing the problem of his physical fighting. One solution generated during the brainstorming session was that he could take karate lessons in order to develop self-control. His parents did not feel that they could evaluate this solution as positive or negative until they learned more about a variety of issues such as the cost of lessons, the location of a karate school, the time that lessons would be scheduled, and so forth. Therefore, as part of their homework for that week, one member of the family took on the responsibility for gathering data about karate schools in the community. The family was then able to evaluate that particular proposed solution at their next session.

## Homework

If the problem-solving discussion was not completed during the session, the family should complete it at home.

Implement any solutions that have been agreed upon.

Each family member should monitor him/herself for negative communication styles. The handout should be posted in a prominent spot in the home, or each family member should take his/her own individual copy. Follow the general principles of good communication.

Conduct another problem-solving discussion at home, using the tape recorder and a blank Problem-Solving Worksheet. The handouts on the problem-solving steps and communication habits should be on display during the discussion. Remind the family to focus on using effective communication styles during this exercise since that is what you will be listening for when you review the tape.

# Practicing Communication Skills

## *Goals*

1. To review problem discussion/communication assignment.
2. To review solution implementations.
3. To continue to practice new communication skills.

## *Materials Required*

- Blank Problem-Solving Worksheet for discussion of homework

## *Session Outline*

- Review homework.
- Continue to practice the steps to better problem solving.
- Continue to practice improving communication habits.

## *Homework*

- Implement agreed-upon solutions.
- Tape record a problem-solving discussion.
- Pay attention to communication styles at any time there is conflict at home.

Question the family concerning the homework assignment. Discuss problems encountered in self-monitoring communication styles during the homework discussion. Were any changes noted in communication styles of each member by other family members? Praise those who improved.

Give the family feedback from the last taped home discussion. Collect this week's tape. If the family is not doing their homework, make this the topic of a problem-solving discussion now.

Review with the family how any previous solutions have worked out over the past week. Discuss any modifications needed. Revisit any problems that are not responding successfully to agreed-upon solutions.

Select a moderately intense problem from the Issues Checklist for problem solving during today's session. Again, pay particular attention to poor communication habits and interrupt the discussion if necessary to instruct family members about using alternative, positive communication skills.

## Common Family Reactions

As the in-session discussions get more heated, and as you begin to address problematic communication styles, the danger arises that the teen will direct his anger or frustration toward you. This must not be tolerated. As the family works on improving communication styles, problems may still arise, with the teen swearing at parents or using disrespectful language toward them in the sessions. This is what they are there to work on, and it should be corrected as it occurs. However, if the teen is disrespectful or swears at the therapist, he/she is to be given one warning and then told to leave the office if it happens again. The parents may remain for the rest of the session (you can address their feelings about their teen's behavior and how it affects them at home) while the teen sits in the waiting room or in the car.

## Homework

Implement solution generated during today's session. Select a problem from the Issues Checklist for discussion at home with the tape recorder.

# Dealing with Unreasonable Beliefs and Expectations

### Goals

1. To review implementation of last week's solution.
2. To give feedback on taped homework discussion.
3. To introduce concept of irrational beliefs separately to the parents and the teens.

### Materials Required

- Parent Handout for Step 15

  Unreasonable Beliefs Chart (keep this chart on display during each session for the remainder of the program)
  Unreasonable and Reasonable Beliefs
- Adolescent Handout for Step 15

  Unreasonable and Reasonable Beliefs
- Blank Problem-Solving Worksheet for homework

### Session Outline

- Review homework.
- Introduce the role of belief systems and expectations.
- Continue to practice the steps to better problem solving.

### Homework

- Family members individually address unreasonable beliefs.
- Conduct a problem-solving discussion.

Review homework and the success or failure of implementing agreed-upon solutions. Give feedback on last week's homework tape.

## The Role of Beliefs Systems and Expectations

After living with defiant teens for as many years as they have, it is easy for parents to begin to "think the worst," and attribute their adolescent's behavior to malicious motives. Because the teens disobey so many rules and argue so incessantly, many parents come to believe that if they give their teenagers more freedom, the teenager will inevitably make serious mistakes and ruin his or her life. In the extreme, we call such thinking *ruination*. Although this occasionally may be true, typically it is an exaggeration that can become a self-fulfilling prophecy: adolescents who believe that their parents always think the worst may misbehave because they figure "they are damned if they do and damned if they don't."

In addition, when the adolescent (inevitably) makes poor decisions or acts coercively, some parents consistently attribute these actions to *malicious intent*—that is, their adolescent is misbehaving on purpose to annoy or anger them. Other parents have lifelong expectations that their children should always *obey* them, and when their children enter adolescence and become more disobedient, such parents respond in a highly punitive manner, spurring rapid escalation of defiant behavior. These expectations for obedience are often part of a more general parental belief that the adolescent should instinctively know how to behave *perfectly*, and that it is catastrophic if he/she doesn't. The teen (let's say a boy) should clean up his room perfectly; he should greet his parents with a smile and a hug; he should look forward to going to visit relatives on the weekend; and he should always get all of his homework done without needing any monitoring. Such perfectionist beliefs are simply not realistic, and are particularly unrealistic for teenagers with ADHD.

Some parents also have unrealistic expectations and beliefs about *love* and *appreciation*. They expect their teenagers to appreciate everything they do for them, which is very rare, and even unnatural, for teenagers. They also believe that they will win their teenagers' affection and obedience by over-indulging them and giving them large gifts and money, whereas they will actually end up reinforcing manipulative and demanding behavior in this manner.

We find that extreme thinking along the themes of ruination, malicious intent, obedience, perfectionism, and love/appreciation adds fuel to the fire of defiance and considerably worsens family conflict. Individuals who adhere rigidly to absolutist beliefs will have a difficult time consistently and dispassionately applying behavior-management and problem-solving techniques. In fact, they may resist implementing these techniques. Thus, one important goal of the second portion of this treatment program is to identify extreme thinking and help modify it.

Adolescents may also adhere to extreme beliefs, which need to be addressed. Most commonly, adolescents adhere to the "unfairness triad" of beliefs: ruination, unfairness, and autonomy. *Unfairness* refers to the belief that parental rules are intrinsically unfair and arbitrary; *ruination* refers to the belief that parental rules will ruin all of the teenager's fun; and *autonomy* refers to the belief that the adolescent should have total and complete freedom from parental restrictions. Teenagers who adhere rigidly to these beliefs experience more conflict with their parents than teens whose expectations are more flexible (Robin, Koepke, & Moye, 1990).

Since parents and adolescents do adhere to somewhat different unreasonable beliefs and expectations, the therapist may decide to divide the session into two portions and deal separately with the parents and adolescents regarding beliefs. Alternatively, as long as the adolescent is not too restless and disruptive, the beliefs can be dealt with in a family session.

## Addressing Unreasonable Beliefs

In this portion of the session, present the rationale for cognitive restructuring, review the most common unreasonable beliefs, identify which ones apply to the parents and adolescent, and help them begin to develop more reasonable beliefs and expectations. Ask the family to engage in the following mental imagery exercise to help them appreciate the connection between extreme thinking, negative affect, and behavioral overreactions (change "son" to "daughter" where appropriate):

"Close your eyes and imagine that you are opening the mail and you find a progress report from your son's school. The progress report indicates that he is failing English and math and has 15 late assignments in history. Suddenly you can feel your blood begin to boil and the tension mount throughout your body. Your son lied to you again!!! He said he was up to date on homework and was passing all of his courses. This is one more example of irresponsible behavior. He is always irresponsible. You told him to keep an assignment book and get help from the teachers. He never does what he is told. He is so disobedient. If he keeps on going this way in school, he is going to fail. He will never graduate, never go to college, and never get a good job. You will be supporting him until the day you die. And the thought of confronting him is not appealing at all. He will deny it at first, then blame it on the teachers, showing you total disrespect. He is just doing this to get you mad and upset. He has no consideration for your feelings. [To the parents] now open your eyes and tell me how you feel and what you are thinking. And also, tell me how you would react if your son walked through the door at this very moment. [To the teen] consider how you think your parents would react in this situation."

Through a Socratic discussion, the therapist helps the parents realize how the extreme thinking evokes extreme affect, and how difficult it would be to deal with the adolescent rationally, as a principle-centered parent is advised to do, in such a strong state of negative affect. Afterward, we suggest to the parents that they strive toward adherence to the following overall coping expectation: "We will encourage our adolescent with ADHD to go for the stars, to do his/her best, but we will accept that it is not a catastrophe when he/she fails to achieve perfection, and it does not mean that he/she is headed for certain ruin or that he/she is purposefully trying to anger us."

After discussing this rationale and the more positive coping attitude, we then distribute copies of the parent and adolescent Unreasonable and Reasonable Beliefs Handouts. We review the examples of common unreasonable beliefs (in the left-hand column), first with the parents and then with the adolescent. As we go through each unreasonable belief, we ask the parents to rate their own adherence to this belief and ask them for examples of particular situations that activated the belief. We look at the reasonable alternative beliefs and expectations (in the right-hand column) and ask the parents and adolescent whether they find them credible. If they do find the reasonable beliefs credible, we continue; otherwise, we review the evidence for the unreasonable versus reasonable belief and suggest experiments the parents can use to test this evidence on their own when the session is over. The therapist does not usually have time to review every belief; one may quickly survey the table and concentrate on the beliefs that seem most salient for a particular family.

The approach to helping family members identify and modify unrealistic expectations and distorted attributions described here can be summarized as follows:

1. Identify the extreme thought.
2. Provide a logical challenge to the extreme thought.
3. Help the family member identify an alternative, more realistic thought.
4. Help the family member collect evidence to disconfirm the extreme thought and confirm the more reasonable thought.

If time permits, after reviewing the handout, help the family identify one irrational belief (either a parental belief or a teen belief) that has led to angry feelings and conflict between family members. This discussion may actually take up the remainder of the session if the family is able to acknowledge these types of scenarios successfully. For some families, however, this topic may seem quite abstract, and it will be the therapist's responsibility to assist those families to understand the concept and experience an "in vivo" example in the session.

If time permits, have the family choose a moderate to intense problem from the Issues Checklist for problem solving in the session. Families may want to add problem topics to the list at this point, since there may be highly conflictual topics that are more unique to a particular family and not covered by the Issues Checklist.

## Common Family Reactions

Irrational beliefs are extremely common for parents. Therefore, as the therapist, you must be able to diplomatically identify these issues for parents in front of the teen in a way that does not undermine the parents' authority. If this does not seem possible for some reason, then it is acceptable to ask the teen to wait in the waiting room for a portion of the session while you have a private discussion with the parents, assisting them to acknowledge the irrationality of certain beliefs or expectations they may hold about their child.

## Homework

Assign for homework the problem solving of an issue that is of at least moderate intensity. As they tape record their discussion, family members may choose to focus on any of their own irrational beliefs that they think might be fueling angry feelings.

You may also wish to give them an assignment to monitor situations in which they adhere to unreasonable expectations or irrational beliefs and to start to challenge these beliefs and expectations.

# Practicing Problem-Solving and Communication Skills: Catching Unreasonable Beliefs

*Goals*

1. To review family's reaction to last week's discussion of unreasonable beliefs.
2. To review implementation of solutions.
3. To continue to practice effective problem solving, improved communication habits, and attention to the impact of beliefs and expectations.

*Materials Required*

- Blank Problem-Solving Worksheet for homework

*Session Outline*

- Discuss homework.
- Discuss a high-intensity problem.

*Homework*

- Conduct a problem-solving discussion practicing all skills learned in the program.

Discuss homework and review any problems in detail. What, if anything, seems to be bogging this family down? Spend as much time as needed on the issues affecting compliance and success with the methods of the program. Review your feedback from the last homework tape. Review the family's reaction to the discussion of unreasonable beliefs, did they identify anything in themselves over the course of the week?

Select an intense, highly conflictual topic for the problem-solving discussion. Focus intensively on "cooling off" in order to avoid using negative communication habits. Identify any possible unreasonable beliefs or expectations that may be fueling the conflict.

## Common Family Reactions

As the end of the program approaches, some families may begin to feel a sense of hopelessness if they do not perceive considerable progress. The therapist will need to focus on the positives in any small gains the parents or the teen have made, emphasizing that it has taken them years to get to this point, and it is probably an "irrational belief" to expect that some of the biggest problems will be solved right away. Encourage families to build on small successes. However, if there are clear roadblocks to success (such as unaddressed parental pathology, an uncooperative school system, lack of community support, or family isolation), then families will benefit from an honest appraisal of these issues and perhaps a problem-solving discussion aimed at taking bigger steps, such as political action, starting a support group, and the like. Some parents, however, may need to mourn their loss of hope that family therapy would solve all their problems.

Some families will report crises that occur and may benefit from specific instructions in how to deal with these crises as they begin to work on their most intense issues. The following suggestions for crisis management have proven clinically useful:

1. Ask the family to describe the types of crisis situations that they encounter. Mention any crises that you observed them to have earlier throughout the therapy. Pinpoint the sequence of escalating affect and try to identify the points at which various family members lose control. What are the triggers for loss of control?
2. Explain that at the time of a crisis, it is best to calm down first and then try to resolve the problem later on.
3. Incorporate anger-management techniques into the remainder of the discussion of crisis management.
4. Identify behavioral and cognitive "stop responses" that would permit family members to keep from "losing it" as the crisis escalates. Examples might include counting to 10, leaving the scene, calling a time out, using calming language, and so forth. Get a commitment from each family member to try to use one of these stop responses.
5. Identify affect-dissipating responses that could take the edge off of family members' anger during a crisis. These might include relaxation training, meditation, mental distraction, physical exercise, punching a pillow, and the like. Get a commitment from each family member to try to use one of these affect-dissipating responses.

6. Role-play a mock crisis, asking family members to use the stop responses and affect-dissipating techniques.
7. Ask them to try the crisis-management techniques at home and report back to you.

## Homework

Select a topic for the taped homework discussion. Implement any solutions generated in today's session. Use crisis-management techniques as needed.

# More Family Practice

*Goals*

1. To review homework.
2. To have a problem-solving discussion of the most difficult issues.

*Materials Required*

- Blank Problem-Solving Worksheet for taped homework discussion

Review homework, solution implementation, and tape from last week. Discuss any roadblocks to success, poor communication habits, or noncompliance with the program.

Address the most intense, conflictual issue on the family's Issues Checklist, utilizing all the problem-solving steps and skills learned about constructive communication habits. Try to step back and let the family handle the discussion as much as possible.

## Common Family Reactions

For some families, all the hot topics have been covered already. If this is the case, you may choose to problem solve "topics" rather than "problems." For example, there may not be a problem yet about independent care of laundry because the teen has not yet gone off to college, but this could be a topic of discussion, with problem solving centering around how to develop these skills. Many teens will welcome the opportunity to do a bit of problem solving in advance of an issue that might be somewhat anxiety provoking.

# Homework

Select a topic for the last taped discussion at home. Remind the family to return the tape recorder (if it is borrowed from you) at the next session (returning their deposit if necessary). Implement any solutions generated during today's session.

# Concluding Treatment

## Goals

1. To review homework.
2. To review any problems that still need to be addressed.
3. To review the major elements of the program.
4. To get family feedback about the program.
5. To establish how to obtain follow-up services if necessary, or schedule a booster session in one month's time for a review of the family's status.

## Materials Required

- Blank Problem-Solving Worksheets if the family would like some

Review the homework discussion. Review any implementation of proposed solutions. Review last week's tape. Praise family for their utilization of skills learned. Review just how far they have come in treatment. Point out their successes.

Help the family to make a plan for how they will address any problems that remain unresolved, providing them with more blank worksheets if they wish.

Review the definitions of ADHD and oppositional behavior, the elements of contingency management and the behavioral contracts, the problem-solving and negotiating steps, and improved communications skills, with emphasis on those issues that have been particularly salient to this family.

Ask the family for feedback about the program, and perhaps have them fill out a patient satisfaction form if your agency collects such data.

Let the family know how they can contact you in the future and what services are available to them in the community.

Say good-bye and congratulations for completing the program!

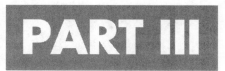

# Assessment Materials

The following instruments are to be used in the evaluation of adolescents referred to mental health professionals when defiant, oppositional, or disruptive behaviors are a major concern. Instructions for the use of these instruments are to be found in Part I of this manual. The General Instructions for Completing the Questionnaires (Form 1) and the Developmental and Medical History Form (Form 3) were initially developed in collaboration with our former colleagues in the ADHD Clinic at the University of Massachusetts Medical Center: Arthur Anastopoulos, PhD, George DuPaul, PhD, and Terri Shelton, PhD. The Clinical Interview—Parent Report Form (Form 6) found here is adapted from the clinical interview found in Barkley's text on defiant children (Barkley, 1997). The other rating scales were developed by Barkley for that same textbook, with the exception of the Issues Checklist, which was originally developed by Robin and Foster (1989).

The author and publisher grant permission to the purchaser of this manual to photocopy these assessment materials solely for use in the purchaser's professional practice and solely for the evaluation of children under the professional care of the purchaser (see the copyright page for details).

## Contents of Part III

General Instructions for Completing the Questionnaires (Form 1)           160

Child and Family Information Form (Form 2)           162

Developmental and Medical History Form (Form 3)           163

Disruptive Behavior Disorders Rating Scale—Parent Form (Form 4)           166

Disruptive Behavior Disorders Rating Scale—Teacher Form (Form 5)           168

Clinical Interview—Parent Report Form (Form 6)           169

Adult Behavior Rating Scale—Self-Report of Current Behavior (Form 7)           194

Adult Behavior Rating Scale—Self-Report of Childhood Behavior (Form 8)           195

Issues Checklist for Parents and Teenagers (Form 9)           196

# GENERAL INSTRUCTIONS FOR COMPLETING THE QUESTIONNAIRES (FORM 1)

In preparation for your teenager's evaluation at our clinic, we ask that you please complete the enclosed forms about your teenager and your family. Your answers will give us a much better understanding of your teen's behavior at home and your family circumstances. In completing these forms, please follow these instructions as closely as possible:

1. *All* forms in this packet should be completed by the parent who has the primary responsibility for caring for this teenager. When both parents reside with the teen, the parent who spends the greatest amount of time with the teen should complete them.

2. If a second parent wishes to complete a second packet of information about the teen, he or she may do so independently by requesting a second set of these forms from our administrative assistant, _____, at _____ (phone) and it will be sent out promptly.

3. If your teenager is currently taking medication for behavioral or emotional problems (such as Ritalin or an antidepressant), we must ask that you complete the questionnaires about your teen's behavior *based on how your teen behaves when* **off** *this medication.* However, some parents whose teens have been on medication for a long time may not be able to give us this information. In that case, just complete the questionnaires based on your teen's current behavior, but check the appropriate line below to let us know that your judgment is of your teen on medication. Check one of the blanks below to let us know for certain on what basis you judged your teenager's behavior in answering our behavior questionnaires:

_____ My teenager currently does *not* take any medication for behavior problems. My answers are based on my teen's behavior while he or she is off of medication.

_____ My teen *is currently taking medication* for behavior problems. However, my answers are based on my teen's behavior while he or she is *off* of this medication.

_____ My teen *is currently taking medication* for behavior problems. My answers are based on my child's behavior while he or she is *on* this medication.

If your teenager is currently taking medication for his or her behavioral or emotional difficulties, please list those medications below, briefly note the reason(s) for their use, and let us know the physician who is prescribing these medications for your teen:

Type of medication: _____

*(cont.)*

Reason for the use of this medication: _____

Physician prescribing this medication is: _____

Thank you for completing these forms and returning them promptly to us in the enclosed envelope.

PLEASE RETURN THIS FORM ALONG WITH THE COMPLETED QUESTIONNAIRES.

# CHILD AND FAMILY INFORMATION (FORM 2)

**Child's name** _____ **Birthdate** _____ **Age** _____

Address _____
              (Street)                       (City)          (State)     (Zip)

Home phone ( ___ ) _____ Work phone ( ___ ) _____ Dad/Mom
                                                                    (Circle one)

Child's school _____ Teacher's name _____

School address _____
                (Street)                      (City)         (State)     (Zip)

School phone ( ___ ) _____ Child's grade _____

Is child in special education?  Yes  No  If so, what type? _____


Father's name _____ Age _____ Education _____
                                                                                    (Years)

Father's place of employment _____

Type of employment _____ Annual salary _____

Mother's name _____ Age _____ Education _____
                                                                                     (Years)

Mother's place of employment _____

Type of employment _____ Annual salary _____

Is child adopted?  Yes  No  If yes, age when adopted_____

Are parents married?  Yes  No  Separated?  Yes  No  Divorced?  Yes  No

Child's physician _____

Physician's address_____
                (Street)                    (City)         (State)     (Zip)

Physician's telephone number_____


Please list all other children in the family:

| Name | Age | School grade |
|------|-----|--------------|
| _____ | _____ | _____ |
| _____ | _____ | _____ |
| _____ | _____ | _____ |
| _____ | _____ | _____ |
| _____ | _____ | _____ |

# DEVELOPMENTAL AND MEDICAL HISTORY (FORM 3)

## PREGNANCY AND DELIVERY

A. Length of pregnancy (e.g., full term, 40 weeks, 32 weeks, etc.)  _____

B. Length of delivery (number of hours from initial labor pains to birth)  _____

C. Mother's age when child was born  _____

D. Child's birth weight  _____

E. Did any of the following conditions occur during pregnancy/delivery?

| | | |
|---|---|---|
| 1. Bleeding | No | Yes |
| 2. Excessive weight gain (more than 30 lbs.) | No | Yes |
| 3. Toxemia/preeclampsia | No | Yes |
| 4. Rh factor incompatibility | No | Yes |
| 5. Frequent nausea or vomiting | No | Yes |
| 6. Serious illness or injury | No | Yes |
| 7. Took prescription medications<br>   a. If yes, name of medication _____ | No | Yes |
| 8. Took illegal drugs | No | Yes |
| 9. Used alcoholic beverage<br>   a. If yes, approximate number of drinks per week ____ | No | Yes |
| 10. Smoked cigarettes<br>   a. If yes, approximate number of cigarettes per day<br>   (e.g., ½ pack) _____ | No | Yes |
| 11. Was given medication to ease labor pains<br>   a. If yes, name of medication _____ | No | Yes |
| 12. Delivery was induced | No | Yes |
| 13. Forceps were used during delivery | No | Yes |
| 14. Had a breech delivery | No | Yes |
| 15. Had a cesarean section delivery | No | Yes |
| 16. Other problems—please describe _____ | No | Yes |

F. Did any of the following conditions affect your child
during delivery or within the first few days after birth?

| | | |
|---|---|---|
| 1. Injured during delivery | No | Yes |
| 2. Cardiopulmonary distress during delivery | No | Yes |

(cont.)

| | | |
|---|---|---|
| 3. Delivered with cord around neck | No | Yes |
| 4. Had trouble breathing following delivery | No | Yes |
| 5. Needed oxygen | No | Yes |
| 6. Was cyanotic, turned blue | No | Yes |
| 7. Was jaundiced, turned yellow | No | Yes |
| 8. Had an infection | No | Yes |
| 9. Had seizures | No | Yes |
| 10. Was given medications | No | Yes |
| 11. Born with a congenital defect | No | Yes |
| 12. Was in hospital more than 7 days | No | Yes |

## INFANT HEALTH AND TEMPERAMENT

A. During the first 12 months, was your child:

| | | |
|---|---|---|
| 1. Difficult to feed | No | Yes |
| 2. Difficult to get to sleep | No | Yes |
| 3. Colicky | No | Yes |
| 4. Difficult to put on a schedule | No | Yes |
| 5. Alert | No | Yes |
| 6. Cheerful | No | Yes |
| 7. Affectionate | No | Yes |
| 8. Sociable | No | Yes |
| 9. Easy to comfort | No | Yes |
| 10. Difficult to keep busy | No | Yes |
| 11. Overactive, in constant motion | No | Yes |
| 12. Very stubborn, challenging | No | Yes |

## EARLY DEVELOPMENTAL MILESTONES

A. At what age did your child first accomplish the following:
1. Sitting without help _____
2. Crawling _____
3. Walking alone, without assistance _____
4. Using single words (e.g.,"mama," "dada," "ball," etc.) _____
5. Putting two or more words together (e.g.,"mama up") _____

(cont.)

6. Bowel training, day and night                                      _____
7. Bladder training, day and night                                    _____

## HEALTH HISTORY

A. Date of child's last physical exam: _____

B. At any time has your child had the following:

| | | | |
|---|---|---|---|
| 1. Asthma | Never | Past | Present |
| 2. Allergies | Never | Past | Present |
| 3. Diabetes, arthritis, or other chronic illnesses | Never | Past | Present |
| 4. Epilepsy or seizure disorder | Never | Past | Present |
| 5. Febrile seizures | Never | Past | Present |
| 6. Chicken pox or other common childhood illnesses | Never | Past | Present |
| 7. Heart or blood pressure problems | Never | Past | Present |
| 8. High fevers (over 103°) | Never | Past | Present |
| 9. Broken bones | Never | Past | Present |
| 10. Severe cuts requiring stitches | Never | Past | Present |
| 11. Head injury with loss of consciousness | Never | Past | Present |
| 12. Lead poisoning | Never | Past | Present |
| 13. Surgery | Never | Past | Present |
| 14. Lengthy hospitalization | Never | Past | Present |
| 15. Speech or language problems | Never | Past | Present |
| 16. Chronic ear infections | Never | Past | Present |
| 17. Hearing difficulties | Never | Past | Present |
| 18. Eye or vision problems | Never | Past | Present |
| 19. Fine motor/handwriting problems | Never | Past | Present |
| 20. Gross motor difficulties, clumsiness | Never | Past | Present |
| 21. Appetite problems (overeating or undereating) | Never | Past | Present |
| 22. Sleep problems (falling asleep, staying asleep) | Never | Past | Present |
| 23. Soiling problems | Never | Past | Present |
| 24. Wetting problems | Never | Past | Present |

25. Other health difficulties—please describe

# DISRUPTIVE BEHAVIOR DISORDERS RATING SCALE—PARENT FORM (FORM 4)

Child's name_____ Age_____ Date_____

Form completed by _____

Relationship to child: [*Circle one*]

    Mother   Father   Stepparent   Other:_____ (explain)

**Instructions:** Circle the number that *best describes* your child's behavior at home over the past 6 months.

| | Never or rarely | Sometimes | Often | Very often |
|---|:---:|:---:|:---:|:---:|
| 1. Fails to give close attention to details or makes careless mistakes in schoolwork | 0 | 1 | 2 | 3 |
| 2. Has difficulty sustaining attention in tasks or play activities | 0 | 1 | 2 | 3 |
| 3. Does not seem to listen when spoken to directly | 0 | 1 | 2 | 3 |
| 4. Does not follow through on instructions and fails to finish work | 0 | 1 | 2 | 3 |
| 5. Has difficulty organizing tasks and activities | 0 | 1 | 2 | 3 |
| 6. Avoids tasks (e.g., schoolwork, homework) that require mental effort | 0 | 1 | 2 | 3 |
| 7. Loses things necessary for tasks or activities | 0 | 1 | 2 | 3 |
| 8. Is easily distracted | 0 | 1 | 2 | 3 |
| 9. Is forgetful in daily activities | 0 | 1 | 2 | 3 |
| 10. Fidgets with hands or feet or squirms in seat | 0 | 1 | 2 | 3 |
| 11. Leaves seat in classroom or in other situations in which remaining seated is expected | 0 | 1 | 2 | 3 |
| 12. Runs about or climbs excessively in situations in which it is inappropriate | 0 | 1 | 2 | 3 |
| 13. Has difficulty playing or engaging in leisure activities quietly | 0 | 1 | 2 | 3 |
| 14. Is "on the go" or acts as if "driven by a motor" | 0 | 1 | 2 | 3 |
| 15. Talks excessively | 0 | 1 | 2 | 3 |
| 16. Blurts out answers before questions have been completed | 0 | 1 | 2 | 3 |
| 17. Has difficulty awaiting turn | 0 | 1 | 2 | 3 |

*(cont.)*

| | Never or rarely | Sometimes | Often | Very often |
|---|---|---|---|---|
| 18. Interrupts or intrudes on others | 0 | 1 | 2 | 3 |
| 19. Loses temper | 0 | 1 | 2 | 3 |
| 20. Argues with adults | 0 | 1 | 2 | 3 |
| 21. Actively defies or refuses to comply with adults' requests or rules | 0 | 1 | 2 | 3 |
| 22. Deliberately annoys people | 0 | 1 | 2 | 3 |
| 23. Blames others for his/her mistakes or misbehavior | 0 | 1 | 2 | 3 |
| 24. Is touchy or easily annoyed by others | 0 | 1 | 2 | 3 |
| 25. Is angry and resentful | 0 | 1 | 2 | 3 |
| 26. Is spiteful or vindictive | 0 | 1 | 2 | 3 |

**Instructions:** Please indicate whether your child has done any of these activities in the past 12 months.

| | | |
|---|---|---|
| 1. Often bullied, threatened, or intimidated others | No | Yes |
| 2. Often initiated physical fights | No | Yes |
| 3. Used a weapon that can cause serious physical harm to others (e.g., a bat, brick, broken bottle, knife, or gun) | No | Yes |
| 4. Has been physically cruel to people | No | Yes |
| 5. Has been physically cruel to animals | No | Yes |
| 6. Has stolen while confronting a victim (e.g., mugging, purse snatching, extortion, armed robbery) | No | Yes |
| 7. Has forced someone into sexual activity | No | Yes |
| 8. Has deliberately engaged in fire setting with the intention of causing serious damage | No | Yes |
| 9. Has deliberately destroyed others' property (other than by fire setting) | No | Yes |
| 10. Has broken into someone else's house, building, or car | No | Yes |
| 11. Often lies to obtain goods or favors or to avoid obligations (i.e., "cons" others) | No | Yes |
| 12. Has stolen items of nontrivial value without confronting a victim (e.g., shoplifting, but without breaking and entering; forgery) | No | Yes |
| 13. Often stays out at night despite parental prohibitions<br>If so, at what age did this begin?____ | No | Yes |
| 14. Has run away from home overnight at least twice while living in parent's home, foster care, or group home.<br>If so, how many times?____ | No | Yes |
| 15. Is often truant from school<br>If so, at what age did he/she begin doing this?____ | No | Yes |

# DISRUPTIVE BEHAVIOR DISORDERS RATING SCALE—TEACHER FORM (FORM 5)

Child's name_____ Date _____

Form completed by _____

Approximately how many hours are you with this child each school day?_____

What subject(s) do you regularly teach this child? _____

**Instructions:** Circle the number that *best describes* this child's behavior at school during the past 6 months.

| | Never or rarely | Sometimes | Often | Very often |
|---|---|---|---|---|
| 1. Fails to give close attention to details or makes careless mistakes in schoolwork | 0 | 1 | 2 | 3 |
| 2. Has difficulty sustaining attention in tasks or play activities | 0 | 1 | 2 | 3 |
| 3. Does not seem to listen when spoken to directly | 0 | 1 | 2 | 3 |
| 4. Does not follow through on instructions and fails to finish work | 0 | 1 | 2 | 3 |
| 5. Has difficulty organizing tasks and activities | 0 | 1 | 2 | 3 |
| 6. Avoids tasks (e.g., schoolwork, homework) that require mental effort | 0 | 1 | 2 | 3 |
| 7. Loses things necessary for tasks or activities | 0 | 1 | 2 | 3 |
| 8. Is easily distracted | 0 | 1 | 2 | 3 |
| 9. Is forgetful in daily activities | 0 | 1 | 2 | 3 |
| 10. Fidgets with hands or feet or squirms in seat | 0 | 1 | 2 | 3 |
| 11. Leaves seat in classroom or in other situations in which remaining seated is expected | 0 | 1 | 2 | 3 |
| 12. Runs about or climbs excessively in situations in which it is inappropriate | 0 | 1 | 2 | 3 |
| 13. Has difficulty playing or engaging in leisure activities quietly | 0 | 1 | 2 | 3 |
| 14. Is "on the go" or acts as if "driven by a motor" | 0 | 1 | 2 | 3 |
| 15. Talks excessively | 0 | 1 | 2 | 3 |
| 16. Blurts out answers before questions have been completed | 0 | 1 | 2 | 3 |
| 17. Has difficulty awaiting turn | 0 | 1 | 2 | 3 |
| 18. Interrupts or intrudes on others | 0 | 1 | 2 | 3 |
| 19. Loses temper | 0 | 1 | 2 | 3 |
| 20. Argues with adults | 0 | 1 | 2 | 3 |
| 21. Actively defies or refuses to comply with adults' requests or rules | 0 | 1 | 2 | 3 |
| 22. Deliberately annoys people | 0 | 1 | 2 | 3 |
| 23. Blames others for his/her mistakes or misbehavior | 0 | 1 | 2 | 3 |
| 24. Is touchy or easily annoyed by others | 0 | 1 | 2 | 3 |
| 25. Is angry and resentful | 0 | 1 | 2 | 3 |
| 26. Is spiteful or vindictive | 0 | 1 | 2 | 3 |

# CLINICAL INTERVIEW—PARENT REPORT FORM (FORM 6)

**Child's name**_____ **Informant**_____

Informant's relationship to child: [*Circle one*]   Mother   Father   Other:_____

Record/chart #_____ Interviewer_____ Date_____

Child's date of birth_____ Age: Years_____ Months_____

Referral source_____ (e.g., school, physician, etc.)

Does referring person wish a copy of the report from this evaluation?   Yes   No

**Clinical Diagnoses:** [*To be filled in after evaluation is completed*]

1._____ 2._____ 3._____

**Clinical Recommendations:** [*To be briefly listed after evaluation is completed*]

1. _____
2. _____
3. _____
4. _____
5. _____
6. _____
7. _____
8. _____
9. _____
10. _____

## LEGAL DISCLOSURES

[*Interviewer: At the start of the interview, be certain to review any necessary legal disclosures pertinent to your state, county, or other geographic region. For instance, in Massachusetts, we advise parents of the following four issues:*]

1. *Any disclosure of information that indicates a suspicion of child abuse must be reported to state authorities (Department of Social Services).*

(cont.)

2. *Any disclosure of threats of harm to oneself, as in a specific suicide threat, will result in immediate referral to an emergency mental health unit.*
3. *Any disclosure of specific threats to specific individuals will result in notification of those individuals concerning the threat.*
4. *Although the mental health records are confidential, they may be subpoenaed by a judge's order and must be provided to the court if so ordered.*

*Take time now to cover any such issues with the family before proceeding to the remainder of this interview.]*

## FAMILY COMPOSITION

Is this child: _____Your biological child _____Adopted _____Foster child

With which parent does the child live? _____Both _____Mother only _____Father only

_____Neither parent; child lives with _____Grandparent _____In foster care

Do you have legal custody of this child?   Yes   No   [*Interviewer: If No, determine whether or not it is legally advisable or permissible to proceed with this evaluation.*]

Does any other adult live in the home?   Yes   No   If so, who is it?_____

How many children are in the family?_____ How many are still at home?_____

## PARENTAL CONCERNS ABOUT CHILD—REASONS FOR EVALUATION

What are you most concerned about regarding your child that led you to request this evaluation? [*Organize parent's responses under major headings below. Query parents about (1) the specific details of each concern, (2) when it began, (3) how often it occurs or how severe it is, and (4) what they have tried to do so far to deal with it.*]

**Home behavior management problems:**

**Home emotional reaction problems:**

(cont.)

**Developmental delays:** [*If present, consider reviewing with parents the diagnostic criteria for Mental Retardation or other specific developmental disorders such as learning disorders.*]

**School behavior-management problems:**

**School work performance or learning problems:**

**School emotional reaction problems:**

**Social interaction problems with peers:**

**Behavior in the community (outside of home and school):**

**Other concerns:**

Why have you decided to seek this evaluation of your child at this time?

(cont.)

What type of assistance or treatment recommendations do you hope to receive from this evaluation?

Now that you have told me what the main concerns that bring you here today are, as well as what you hope to gain from the evaluation, I need to go over a number of different topics with you about your child. This needs to be done to be sure that I get as comprehensive a picture of your child's psychological adjustment as possible. I am going to ask you about a number of important developmental areas for any child. You should tell me if you have noticed anything unusual, abnormal, atypical, or even bizarre about your child's functioning in any of these areas. Let's begin with your child's:

**Sensory development** (impairments in vision, hearing, sense of touch or smell; abnormal reactions to sensory stimulation; hallucinations, etc.):

**Motor development** (coordination, gait, balance, posture, movements, gestures, tics, nervous habits or mannerisms, etc.):

**Language development** (delays, comprehension problems, speech difficulties):

**Emotional development** (overreactions, mood swings, extreme or unpredictable moods, peculiar or odd emotions, unusual fears or anxieties, etc.):

**Thinking** (odd ideas, bizarre preoccupations or fixations, unusual fantasies, speaks in incomplete or incoherent thoughts, delusions):

(cont.)

**Social behavior** (aggressive, rejected, bullies others, withdrawn, shy, anxious around others, mute when with others, aloof from others or shows no desire for friends/playmates, etc.):




**Intelligence/academic skills** (delays in general mental development; problems with memory; or specific delays in reading, math, spelling, handwriting, or other academic skill areas):




## REVIEW OF DSM-IV CHILDHOOD DISORDERS

Now I need to ask you a number of very specific questions about a variety of behavioral, social, or emotional problems that children sometimes have difficulties with. As I ask you about them, keep in mind that some of these things are not bad or abnormal and may be seen sometimes in healthy, normal children. I want you to tell me if your child does any of these things to a degree that you consider to be inappropriate for someone of his/her age and sex.

[Interviewer: If this child is a member of a minority group in this country or used to reside in a foreign country, be sure to follow up any answer by the parent that endorses a symptom as present with the following question: "Yes, but do you consider this to be a problem or to be inappropriate for a child of your ethnic or cultural group?"]

### Oppositional Defiant Disorder

[Interviewer: Diagnosis requires four or more symptoms. Symptoms must be inappropriate for child's age; must have lasted at least the past 6 months; and must be producing clear evidence of clinically significant impairment in social, academic, or occupational functioning.]

I am now going to ask you some specific questions about your child's behavior during the past 6 months. For each of the behaviors I ask you about, please tell me if your child shows that behavior to a degree that is inappropriate compared to other children of your child's age.

A. Oppositional Defiant List [Enter 1 if present, 0 if absent, and ? if unknown.]

   During the past 6 months, did your child show any of the following:

   1. Often loses temper                                                     ____
   2. Often argues with adults                                               ____

*(cont.)*

Note. The questions in the remainder of this form are adapted from the diagnostic criteria of the DSM-IV (American Psychiatric Association, 1994). Copyright 1994 by the American Psychiatric Association. Adapted by permission.

3. Often actively defies or refuses to comply with adults' requests or rules ____
4. Often deliberately annoys people ____
5. Often blames others for his/her own mistakes or misbehavior ____
6. Is often touchy or easily annoyed by others ____
7. Is often angry or resentful ____
8. Is often spiteful or vindictive ____

B. Have these behaviors existed for at least the past 6 months? [*Enter 1 if present, 0 if absent, and ? if unknown.*] ____

C. At what age did these behaviors first cause problems for your child? ____ (yrs.)

D. Have these behaviors created problems or impairment for your child in either of the following areas? [*Enter 1 if present, 0 if absent, and ? if unknown.*]
Social relations with others ____ Academic performance ____

E. Exclusion Criteria: [*Interviewer: Enter 1 if symptoms occur only during a Psychotic Disorder or Mood Disorder or if criteria are met for Conduct Disorder. Enter 0 if not, ? if unknown.*] ____

*Diagnostic Code*

Requirements for diagnosis:

Does section A total 4 or more? ____
Does section B total 1? ____
Does section D total 1 or more? ____
Does section E total 0? ____

[*Check here if all requirements are met.*]

☐ ODD (313.81)

## Conduct Disorder

[*Interviewer: Diagnosis requires three or more symptoms during previous 12 months and at least one during the past 6 months; the symptoms must presently be causing impairment in social or academic functioning.*]

Now I want to ask you about some other things your child may have done. For these behaviors, I want you to think about the past 12 months and tell me whether any of these have occurred during that time.

A. Conduct Disorder List [*Enter 1 if present, 0 if absent, and ? if unknown.*]
During the past 12 months, did your child do any of the following:

1. Often bullies, threatens, or intimidates others ____
2. Often initiates physical fights ____

*(cont.)*

3. Has used a weapon that can cause serious physical harm to others (e.g., a bat, brick, broken bottle, knife, or gun) _____
4. Has been physically cruel to people _____
5. Has been physically cruel to animals _____
6. Has stolen while confronting a victim (e.g., mugging, purse snatching, extortion, armed robbery) _____
7. Has forced someone into sexual activity _____
8. Has deliberately engaged in fire setting with the intention of causing serious damage _____
9. Has deliberately destroyed others' property (other than by fire setting) _____
10. Has broken into someone else's house, building, or car _____
11. Often lies to obtain goods or favors or to avoid obligations (i.e., "cons" others) _____
12. Has stolen items of nontrivial value without confronting a victim (e.g., shoplifting, but without breaking and entering; forgery) _____
13. Often stays out at night despite parental prohibitions _____
    If so, at what age did this begin? _____ (yrs.)
    [Interviewer: Must begin before age 13 years to be counted as a symptom.]
14. Has run away from home overnight at least twice while living in parent's home, foster care, or group home _____
    If so, how many times? _____
    [Interviewer: Count as a symptom if it occurred once without child returning for a lengthy period.]
15. Is often truant from school _____
    If so, at what age did he/she begin doing this? _____ (yrs.)
    [Interviewer: Must begin before age 13 years to be counted as a symptom.]

B. Have three of these behaviors occurred during the past 12 months? _____
   [Enter 1 if present, 0 if absent, and ? if unknown.]

C. Has at least one of these behaviors occurred during the past 6 months? _____
   [Enter 1 if present, 0 if absent, and ? if unknown.]

D. Did any of these behaviors occur prior to age 10 years? _____
   [Enter 1 if present, 0 if absent, and ? if unknown.]

E. Have these behaviors created problems or impairment for your child in either of the following areas? [Enter 1 if present, 0 if absent, and ? if unknown.]
   Social relations with others _____ Academic performance _____

F. Exclusion Criteria: [Interviewer: Enter 1 if the child is 18 years of age or older and criteria are met for Antisocial Personality Disorder. Enter 0 if not, ? if unknown.] _____

(cont.)

*Diagnostic Code*

Requirements for diagnosis:

Does section A total 3 or more? \_\_\_\_
Does section B total 1? \_\_\_\_
Does section C total 1? \_\_\_\_
Does section E total 1 or more? \_\_\_\_
Does section F total 0? \_\_\_\_

[*Check one subtype if all requirements are met.*]

☐ CD, Childhood-Onset Type (312.8) [*Onset of at least one symptom prior to age 10 years*]
☐ CD, Adolescent-Onset Type (312.8) [*Absence of any symptoms prior to age 10 years*]

*Severity:* [*Check appropriate severity level*]

☐ Mild [*Few, if any, conduct problems in excess of those required to make the diagnosis and conduct problems cause only minor harm to others.*]
☐ Moderate [*Number of conduct problems and effect on others is intermediate between "mild" and "severe."*]
☐ Severe [*Many conduct problems have occurred in excess of those required to make the diagnosis or conduct problems cause considerable harm to others.*]

## Disruptive Behavior Disorder, NOS

[*Interviewer: This category is for disruptive disorders characterized by conduct or oppositional–defiant behaviors that do not meet criteria for CD or ODD but that produce clinically significant impairment.*]

☐ Disruptive Behavior Disorder, NOS (312.9)

## Attention-Deficit/Hyperactivity Disorder

[*Interviewer: Diagnosis requires six Inattention symptoms and/or six Hyperactive–Impulsive symptoms. Symptoms must also be inappropriate for child's age, have lasted at least the past 6 months, and have caused some impairment prior to age 7 years; presently must be causing impairment in two situations (home, school, or work functioning); and must be producing clear evidence of clinically significant impairment in social or academic functioning.*]

Let me ask you about some other behaviors that your child may have shown during the past 6 months. Again, for each of the behaviors I ask you about, please tell me if your child shows that behavior to a degree that is inappropriate compared to other children of your child's age.

A. Inattention List [*Enter 1 if present, 0 if absent, and ? if unknown.*]

During the past 6 months, did your child show any of the following:

1. Often fails to give close attention to details or makes careless mistakes in schoolwork, work, or other activities \_\_\_\_

(cont.)

2. Often has difficulty sustaining attention in tasks or play activities ____

3. Often does not seem to listen when spoken to directly ____

4. Often does not follow through on instructions and fails to finish schoolwork, chores, or duties at work [*Interviewer: Inquire to be sure this is not due solely to oppositional behavior or failure to understand instructions.*] ____

5. Often has difficulty organizing tasks and activities ____

6. Often avoids, dislikes, or is reluctant to engage in tasks that require sustained mental effort (such as schoolwork or homework) ____

7. Often loses things necessary for tasks or activities (e.g., toys, school assignments, pencils, books, or tools) ____

8. Is often easily distracted by extraneous stimuli ____

9. Is often forgetful in daily activities ____

B. Hyperactive–Impulsive List [*Enter 1 if present, 0 if absent, and ? if unknown.*]

During the past 6 months, did your child show any of the following:

1. Often fidgets with hands or feet or squirms in his/her seat ____

2. Often leaves his/her seat in the classroom or in other situations in which remaining seated is expected ____

3. Often runs about or climbs excessively in situations in which it is inappropriate to do so [*Interviewer: For adolescents, this may be limited to subjective feelings of restlessness.*] ____

4. Often has difficulty playing or engaging in leisure activities quietly ____

5. Is often "on the go" or often acts as if "driven by a motor" ____

6. Often talks excessively ____

7. Often blurts out answers before questions have been completed ____

8. Often has difficulty awaiting his/her turn ____

9. Often interrupts or intrudes on others (e.g., butts into conversations or games) ____

C. Have these behaviors existed for at least the past 6 months? ____

[*Enter 1 if present, 0 if absent, and ? if unknown.*]

D. At what age did these behaviors first cause problems for your child? [*Interviewer: Onset by age 13 is acceptable, although DSM-IV stipulates age 7.*] ____ (yrs.)

E. During the past 6 months, have these behaviors caused problems for this child in any of the following situations? [*Enter 1 if present, 0 if absent, and ? if unknown.*]

At home ____ In school ____ At daycare or with babysitters ____

In community activities (clubs, sports, scouts, etc.) ____

F. Have these behaviors created problems or impairment for your child in any of the following areas? [*Enter 1 if present, 0 if absent, and ? if unknown.*]

Social relations with others ____ Academic performance ____

(cont.)

G. Exclusion Criteria: [*Interviewer: Enter 1 if symptoms occur only during a Pervasive Developmental Disorder or Psychotic Disorder or are better accounted for by another mental disorder, such as a Mood, Anxiety, Dissociative, or Personality Disorder. Enter 0 if not, ? if unknown.*] ____

*Diagnostic Code*

    Requirements for diagnosis:

        Does section A total 6 or more, or does section B total 6 or more? ____
        Does section C total 1? ____
        Does section E total 2 or more? ____
        Does section F total 1 or more? ____
        Does section G total 0? ____

    [*Check one subtype if all requirements are met.*]

    ☐ ADHD, Combined Type (314.01) [*Meets criteria for both Inattention and Hyperactive–Impulsive lists*]
    ☐ ADHD, Predominantly Inattentive Type (314.00) [*Meets criteria only for Inattention items*]
    ☐ ADHD, Predominantly Hyperactive–Impulsive Type (314.01) [*Meets criteria only for Hyperactive–Impulsive items*]
    ☐ ADHD, NOS (Not Otherwise Specified) (314.9) [*For disorders with prominent symptoms that do not meet full criteria for any subtype of ADHD*]

For individuals (especially adolescents and adults) who currently have symptoms that no longer meet full criteria, specify "In Partial Remission": _____

## ANXIETY AND MOOD DISORDERS

Now I would like to ask you some questions about your child's emotions in general and his/her emotional reactions to some specific situations. I'll begin by asking you about any specific fears that your child may have. Then I will ask you about his/her general mood or emotional condition throughout much of the day. Let's start with some specific fears that your child may have.

### Specific Phobia

[*Interviewer: Diagnosis requires that each criteria A–F below be met.*]

A. Does your child show a marked and persistent fear that is excessive or unreasonable in response to the presence of or the anticipation of a specific object or situation? For instance, in response to or anticipation of certain animals, heights, being in the dark, thunderstorms or lightning, flying, receiving an injection, seeing blood, or any other things or situations? ____

    [*Enter 1 if present, 0 if absent, and ? if unknown.*]

*(cont.)*

[*Interviewer: If A is present, answer the following, then proceed to B–G below; otherwise, skip to the next disorder. If any of criteria B–F are not met, skip to the next disorder.*]

What specifically is your child fearful of? _____

B.  Does your child have this anxious or fearful reaction almost invariably when exposed to (specific thing or situation)?                                                        ____

[*Enter 1 if present, 0 if absent, and ? if unknown.*]

[*Interviewer: This may include a panic attack in the presence of the feared object or situation; or anxiety expressed by crying, tantrums, freezing, or clinging. Also, children do not need to recognize that their fear is excessive or unreasonable to qualify for this diagnosis.*]

C.  Does your child attempt to avoid this thing or situation, or, if he/she must be exposed to it, does he/she endure it with intense anxiety or distress?                          ____

[*Enter 1 if present, 0 if absent, and ? if unknown.*]

D.  Does your child's avoidance of, anticipation of, or anxious reaction to this thing or situation interfere significantly with any of the following? [*Enter 1 if present, 0 if absent, and ? if unknown.*]

[*Interviewer: Only one of these conditions needs to be endorsed for this criterion to be met.*]

His/her normal routine ____ Academic functioning ____

Social activities ____ Social relationships ____

E.  Does having this fear cause him/her marked distress?                                     ____

F.  Has your child had this fearful or anxious reaction to this thing or event over a period of at least the past 6 months?                                                      ____

[*Enter 1 if present, 0 if absent, and ? if unknown.*]

G.  Exclusion Criteria: [*Interviewer: Enter 1 if this phobia or anxiety is better accounted for by another mental disorder, such as Obsessive–Compulsive Disorder, Posttraumatic Stress Disorder, Separation Anxiety Disorder, Social Phobia, or Panic Disorder. Enter 0 if not, ? if unknown.*]                                                       ____

*Diagnostic Code*

Requirements for diagnosis:

Do each of sections A through F total 1 or more?  ____
Does section G total 0?  ____

[*Check here if all requirements are met.*]

☐ Specific Phobia (300.29)

## Social Phobia

[*Interviewer: Diagnosis requires that each criteria A–F below be met, but the child must have developed the capacity for age-appropriate social relationships with familiar people and the anxiety must occur in peer settings, not just in interactions with adults.*]

(cont.)

What about social situations?

A. [*Enter 1 if present, 0 if absent, and ? if unknown.*]

   1. Does your child show a marked and persistent fear that is excessive or unreasonable in response to the presence of or the anticipation of a social or performance situation in which he/she is exposed to unfamiliar people or to possible scrutiny by others? \_\_\_\_

   2. Does your child fear that he/she will act in a way that will be embarrassing or humiliating or will be so anxious that it will be humiliating or embarrassing for him/her? \_\_\_\_
   [*Interviewer: If parts 1 and 2 of A are present, answer the next question and then proceed with remaining criteria below; otherwise, skip to the next disorder. If any of the remaining criteria below are not met, skip to the next disorder.*]

   3. What specific social situation is your child fearful of? _____

B. Does your child have this anxious or fearful reaction almost invariably when exposed to this situation? \_\_\_\_

   [*Enter 1 if present, 0 if absent, and ? if unknown.*]

   [*Interviewer: This may include a panic attack in this social situation or anxiety expressed by crying, tantrums, freezing, clinging, or shrinking from this social situation with unfamiliar people. Also, children do not need to recognize that their fear is excessive or unreasonable to qualify for this diagnosis.*]

C. Does your child attempt to avoid this situation or, if he/she must be exposed to it, does he/she endure it with intense anxiety or distress? \_\_\_\_

   [*Enter 1 if present, 0 if absent, and ? if unknown.*]

D. Does your child's avoidance of, anticipation of, or anxious reaction to this situation interfere significantly with any of the following? [*Enter 1 if present, 0 if absent, and ? if unknown.*]

   [*Interviewer: Only one of these conditions needs to be endorsed for this criterion to be met.*]

   His/her normal routine \_\_\_\_ Academic functioning \_\_\_\_

   Social activities \_\_\_\_ Social relationships \_\_\_\_

E. Does having this fear cause him/her marked distress? \_\_\_\_

F. Has your child had this fearful or anxious reaction to this situation for at least the past 6 months? \_\_\_\_

   [*Enter 1 if present, 0 if absent, and ? if unknown.*]

G. Exclusion Criteria: [*Interviewer: Enter 1 if this phobia or anxiety is due to the direct physiological effects of a substance or a general medical condition, or is not better accounted for by another mental disorder, such as Panic Disorder, Separation Anxiety Disorder, Body Dysmorphic Disorder, Pervasive Developmental Disorder, or Schizoid Personality Disorder. Or, if a general medical condition or another mental disorder is present, enter 1 if the fear in Criterion A above is related to it. Enter 0 if not, ? if unknown.*] \_\_\_\_

(cont.)

*Diagnostic Code*

Requirements for diagnosis:

Does section A total 2? ____
Does each section B through F equal 1 or more? ____
Does section G total 0? ____

[*Check here if all requirements are met.*]

☐ Social Phobia (300.23)
Specify if Generalized (fear includes most social situations): _____

## Separation Anxiety Disorder

[*Interviewer: Diagnosis requires that at least three symptoms be present (see A below) for at least 4 weeks. The symptoms must have developed before age 18 years and must produce clinically significant distress or impairment in social, academic, or other important areas of functioning, and other disorders must be excluded, as indicated below.*]

A. Separation Anxiety Disorder Symptom List

Now let's talk about how your child reacts emotionally when he/she must be away from you or when he/she must leave home for activities in the community. Does your child show any of the following? [*Enter 1 if present, 0 if absent, and ? if unknown.*]

1. Recurrent, excessive distress when separation from home, a parent, or a major attachment figure occurs or is anticipated ____

2. Persistent and excessive worry about losing a parent or major attachment figure or about possible harm occurring to such a figure ____

3. Persistent and excessive worry that an unexpected or untoward event will lead him/her to become separated from a parent or major attachment figure (e.g., getting lost or being kidnapped) ____

4. Persistent reluctance or refusal to go to school or elsewhere because of fear of separation ____

5. Persistent and excessive fear or reluctance to be alone, without a parent or major attachment figure at home, or without such a parent or caregiver when in other settings ____

6. Persistent reluctance or refusal to go to sleep without being near a major attachment figure or to sleep away from home ____

7. Repeated nightmares involving the theme or topic of separation from a parent or other caregiver ____

8. Repeated complaints of physical symptoms, such as headaches, stomachaches, nausea, or vomiting, when separation from a parent or major attachment figure occurs or is anticipated ____

[*Interviewer: If three or more symptoms were endorsed, proceed with remaining criteria; otherwise, skip to next disorder. If any of the remaining criteria below are not met, skip to the next disorder.*]

(cont.)

B. Have these fears existed for at least 4 weeks? ____

[*Enter 1 if present, 0 if absent, and ? if unknown.*]

C. At what age did these behaviors first cause problems for your child? ____ (yrs.)

[*Interviewer: Symptoms must have developed before age 18 years.*]

D. Have these worries created distress for your child or impairment in any of the following areas?

[*Enter 1 if present, 0 if absent, and ? if unknown.*]

Social relations with others ____ Academic performance ____

Any other areas of functioning ____

E. Exclusion Criteria: [*Interviewer: Enter 1 if symptoms occur only during a Pervasive Developmental Disorder, Schizophrenia, or other Psychotic Disorder, or are not better accounted for by Panic Disorder. Enter 0 if not, ? if unknown.*] ____

*Diagnostic Code*

Requirements for diagnosis:

Does section A total 3 or more? ____
Does section B total 1? ____
Does section C show 17 years or less? ____
Does section D total 1 or more? ____
Does section E total 0? ____

[*Check here if all requirements are met.*]

☐ Separation Anxiety Disorder (309.21)

Specify if Early Onset (before age 6 years): _____

**Generalized Anxiety Disorder**

[*Interviewer: Diagnosis requires that criteria A and B be met; that at least one symptom in criterion C be present for at least 6 months on more days than not; that symptoms produce clinically significant distress or impairment in social, academic, or other important areas of functioning; and that other disorders be excluded, as indicated below.*]

Now let's talk about whether your child tends to be generally anxious or to worry a lot compared to other children of his/her age group.

A. [*Enter 1 if present, 0 if absent, and ? if unknown.*]

1. Does your child show excessive anxiety and worry about a number of events or activities, such as work activities, school performance, or any other situations? ____

2. Has this anxiety or worry occurred on more days than not for at least the last 6 months? ____

(*cont.*)

*[Interviewer: If the questions in A above were endorsed, proceed with remaining criteria for this disorder; otherwise, skip to next disorder. If any of the remaining criteria below are not met, skip to the next disorder.]*

B. Does your child find it difficult to control his/her worry? ____

C. Generalized Anxiety Disorder Symptom List

Has your child's anxiety or worry been associated with any of the following behaviors for more days than not over the past 6 months? *[Enter 1 if present, 0 if absent, and ? if unknown.]*

*[Interviewer: Only one condition needs to be present for this criterion to be met.]*

1. Restlessness or feeling keyed up or on edge ____
2. Being easily fatigued or tired ____
3. Difficulty concentrating or mind going blank ____
4. Irritability ____
5. Muscle tension ____
6. Sleep disturbance or difficulties falling asleep, staying asleep, or restless and unsatisfying sleep ____

D. Have these worries created distress for your child or impairment in any of the following areas? *[Enter 1 if present, 0 if absent, and ? if unknown.]*

Social relations with others ____ Academic performance ____

Any other areas of functioning ____

E. Exclusion Criteria: *[Interviewer: Enter 1 if the anxiety or worry are confined to features of another mental disorder, such as being worried about having a panic attack (Panic Disorder), being embarrassed in public (Social Phobia), being contaminated (Obsessive–Compulsive Disorder), being away from home or major attachment figures (Separation Anxiety Disorder), having multiple physical complaints (Somatization Disorder), or having a serious illness (Hypochondriasis); or if the anxiety is associated with Posttraumatic Stress Disorder. Also, enter 1 if the disturbance is due to the direct physiological effects of a substance (e.g., drug abuse, medication) or a general medical condition (e.g., hyperthyroidism) or occurs exclusively during a Mood Disorder, a Psychotic Disorder, or a Pervasive Developmental Disorder. Enter 0 if not, ? if unknown.]* ____

*Diagnostic Code*

Requirements for diagnosis:

Does section A total 2? ____
Does section B total 1? ____
Does section C total 1 or more? ____
Does section D total 1 or more? ____
Does section E total 0? ____

*[Check here if all requirements are met.]*

☐ Generalized Anxiety Disorder (300.02)

*(cont.)*

**Dysthymic Disorder**

[*Interviewer: Diagnosis requires that depressed mood exist for most of the day, for more days than not, for at least 1 year; that at least two symptoms from B exist; that the child has never been without the symptoms in A and B below for 2 consecutive months during the 1 year of the disturbance; that all exclusionary criteria are met; and that the symptoms cause clinically significant distress or impairment in social, academic, or other important areas of functioning.*]

I would like to speak with you now about your child's general mood.

A. [*Enter 1 if present, 0 if absent, and ? if unknown.*] Does your child show depressed mood or irritability for most of the day, by either his/her own report or your own observations of your child? ____

Has this depressed mood occurred more days than not for at least the past 12 months? ____

[*Interviewer: If the two questions in A above were endorsed, proceed with remaining criteria for this disorder; otherwise, skip to next disorder. If any of the remaining criteria are not met, skip to the next disorder.*]

B. Does your child show any of the following difficulties while he/she is depressed: [*Enter 1 if present, 0 if absent, and ? if unknown.*]

1. Poor appetite or overeating ____
2. Insomnia (trouble falling asleep) or hypersomnia (excessive sleeping) ____
3. Low energy or fatigue ____
4. Low self-esteem ____
5. Poor concentration or difficulty making decisions ____
6. Feelings of hopelessness ____

C. During the 12 months or more that your child has shown this depressed mood, has he/she ever been without this depressed mood or the other difficulties you mentioned for at least 2 consecutive months? ____

[*Enter 0 if the child has had a 2-month remission, 1 if he/she has not had any remission of symptoms for at least 2 months, and ? if unknown.*]

D. Has this depressed mood created distress for your child or impairment in any of the following areas? [*Enter 1 if present, 0 if absent, and ? if unknown.*]

Social relations with others ____ Academic performance ____

Any other areas of functioning ____

E. Exclusion Criteria: [*Interviewer: Enter 1 if the child meets criteria for Major Depressive Episode during the year or more of his/her mood disorder or if the disorder is better accounted for by Major Depressive Disorder. Also, enter 1 if there has ever been a manic episode, mixed manic–depressive episode, or hypomanic episode; or if criteria for Cyclothymic Disorder apply. Enter 1 if the disorder described above occurs exclusively during the course of a chronic Psychotic Disorder, Schizophrenia, or Delusional Disorder or is the result of the direct physiological effects of a substance or a general medical condition. Enter 0 if not, ? if unknown.*] ____

(cont.)

*Diagnostic Code*

Requirements for diagnosis:

Does section A total 2? ——
Does section B total 2 or more? ——
Does section C total 1? ——
Does section D total 1 or more? ——
Does section E total 0? ——

*[Check here if all requirements are met.]*

☐ Dysthymic Disorder (300.4)

## Major Depressive Disorder

*[Interviewer: Diagnosis requires that at least five or more of the symptoms listed in A below have been present for a 2-week period; that this represents a change from previous functioning; that at least one of the symptoms is depressed mood or loss of interest or pleasure; that the symptoms create clinically significant distress or impairment in social, academic, or other important areas of functioning; and that all exclusion criteria are met.]*

A. Major Depressive Disorder Symptom List

Let's continue to talk about your child's mood or emotional adjustment. Has your child developed any of the following for at least a 2-week period of time? *[Enter 1 if present, 0 if absent, and ? if unknown.]*

1. Depressed or irritable mood most of the day nearly every day for at least 2 weeks ——
   *[This can be by the child's own report or by the parents' or others' observations.]*

2. Markedly diminished interest or pleasure in all or almost all activities most of the day, nearly every day for at least 2 weeks ——
   *[This can be by the child's own report or by the parents' or others' observations.]*
   *[Interviewer: If either 1 or 2 was endorsed, proceed with remaining criteria; otherwise, skip to the next disorder.]*

3. Significant weight loss, when not dieting ——
   Significant weight gain ——
   Decrease or increase in appetite nearly every day ——
   Failed to meet expected weight gains ——

4. Insomnia (trouble falling asleep) or hypersomnia (excessive sleep) nearly every day ——

5. Agitated or excessive movement nearly every day ——
   *[Must be supported by the parents' or others' observations.]*
   Lethargic, sluggish, slow moving, or significantly reduced movement or activity nearly every day ——
   *[Must be supported by the parents' or others' observations.]*

(cont.)

6. Fatigue or loss of energy nearly every day ____

7. Feelings of worthlessness or excessive or inappropriate guilt nearly every day ____
   [*Interviewer: This should not be just self-reproach or guilt about being sick.*]

8. Diminished ability to think or concentrate, or indecisiveness, nearly every day ____
   [*Can be by child's self-report or parent's or others' observations.*]

9. Recurrent thoughts of death ____
   Recurrent thoughts of suicide without a specific plan ____
   Suicide attempt or a specific plan for committing suicide ____

[*Interviewer: If five or more of symptoms 1–9 were endorsed, proceed. If not, skip to the next disorder.*]

B. Have these symptoms of depression created distress for your child or impairment in any of the following areas? [*Enter 1 if present, 0 if absent, and ? if unknown.*]

Social relations with others ____ Academic performance ____

Any other areas of functioning ____

C. Exclusion Criteria: [*Interviewer: Enter 1 if the child meets criteria for Bipolar Disorder; if the symptoms are due to direct physiological effects of a substance or a general medical condition; if the symptoms are better accounted for by clinical Bereavement after the loss of a loved one or by Schizoaffective Disorder; if the symptoms are superimposed on Schizophrenia, Schizophreniform Disorder, Delusional Disorder, or Psychotic Disorder NOS; or if there has been a Manic Episode, a Mixed Episode, or a Hypomanic Episode. Enter 0 if not, ? if unknown.*] ____

*Diagnostic Code*

Requirements for diagnosis:

Do questions 1 and 2 in section A total 1 or more? ____
Does section A total 5 or more? ____
Does section B total 1 or more? ____
Does section C total 0? ____

[*Check here if all requirements are met.*]

☐ Major Depressive Disorder (296.xx)
[*Code for single episode is 296.2x, recurrent episodes is 296.3x; see pp. 344–345 of DSM-IV for additional specifications about the disorder.*]

## Depressive Disorder, NOS

[*Interviewer: Code this only when there is clinically significant depression with impairment, but where full criteria for Major Depressive Disorder, Dysthymic Disorder, Adjustment Disorder with Depressed Mood, or Adjustment Disorder with Mixed Anxiety and Depressed Mood are not met.*]

☐ Depressive Disorder, NOS (311)

*(cont.)*

## Bipolar I Disorder: Manic Episode

[*Interviewer: Diagnosis requires that the child has had a distinct period of at least 1 week of abnormally and persistently elevated, expansive, or irritable mood, or any period of such mood that resulted in hospitalization; and has had at least three of the symptoms listed in B below (or four if mood was primarily irritable) to a significant degree. Also, the symptoms must create clinically significant impairment in social, academic, or other important areas of functioning, and exclusion criteria must be met.*]

I have some more questions to ask you about your child's moods or emotional adjustment.

A. Has your child ever experienced a period of time that lasted at least 1 week: [*Enter 1 if present, 0 if absent, and ? if unknown.*]

1. When his/her mood was unusually and persistently elevated; that is, he/she felt abnormally happy, giddy, joyous, or ecstatic well beyond normal feelings of happiness? _____

2. Or when his/her mood was abnormally and persistently expansive; that is, your child felt able to accomplish everything he/she decided to do, felt nearly super human in his/her ability to do anything he/she wished to do, or felt as if his/her abilities were without limits? _____

3. Or when his/her mood was abnormally and persistently irritable; that is, he/she was unusually touchy, too easily prone to anger or temper outbursts, too easily annoyed by events or by others, or abnormally cranky? _____

[*Interviewer: If any of the above three were endorsed, proceed with B; otherwise, skip to next disorder.*]

B. During the week or more that your child showed this abnormal and persistent mood, did you notice any of the following to be persistent and/or occurring to an abnormal or significant degree? [*Enter 1 if present, 0 if absent, and ? if unknown.*]

1. Had inflated self-esteem or felt grandiose about self well beyond what would be characteristic for his/her level of abilities _____

2. Showed a decreased need for sleep; for instance, he/she stated that he/she felt rested after only 3 hours of sleep _____

3. Was more talkative than usual or seemed to feel pressured to keep talking _____

4. Skipped from one idea to another and then another in speech as if his/her ideas were flying rapidly by _____

   Stated that he/she felt that his/her thoughts were racing or flying by at an abnormal rate of speed _____

5. Was distractible; that is, his/her attention was too easily drawn to unimportant or irrelevant events or things around him/her _____

6. Showed an increase in goal-directed activity; that is, he/she became unusually and persistently productive or directed more activity than normal toward the tasks he/she wanted to accomplish _____

   Seemed very agitated, overly active, or abnormally restless _____

(*cont.*)

7. Showed an excessive involvement in pleasurable activities that have a
   high likelihood of negative, harmful, or painful consequences          ____

[*Interviewer: If three or more symptoms above were endorsed, proceed with remaining criteria; otherwise, skip to next disorder.*]

C. [*Enter 1 if present, 0 if absent, and ? if unknown.*]

1. Was this disturbance in your child's mood enough to cause severe impairment,
   disruption, or difficulties with social relationships, academic performance,
   or other important activities                                          ____

2. Or, did your child's abnormal mood lead to him/her being hospitalized to
   prevent harm to him/herself or others                                 ____

3. Or, did your child have hallucinations (explain) or bizarre ideas
   (psychotic thinking), or feel or act paranoid (as if others were intentionally
   out to harm him/her)                                                   ____

[*Interviewer: If one or more of the criteria 1–3 is endorsed, proceed.*]

D. Exclusion Criteria: [*Interviewer: Enter 1 if the symptoms meet criteria for Mixed Manic–Depressive Episode or Schizoaffective Disorder, are the direct physiological effects of a substance or a general medical condition, or are superimposed on Schizophrenia, Schizophreniform Delusional Disorder, or Psychotic Disorder NOS. Enter 0 if not, ? if unknown. Also, if the child meets criteria for ADHD, enter 0 only if the child meets the criteria after excluding distractibility (5, above) and psychomotor agitation (second part of 6, above).*]  ____

*Diagnostic Code*

Requirements for diagnosis:

Does section A total 1 or more?  ____
Does section B total 3 or more?  ____
Does section C total 1 or more?  ____
Does section D total 0?          ____

[*Check here if all requirements are met.*]

☐ Bipolar I Disorder: Manic Episode (296.xx)
[*Code 296.0x if single episode; 296.40 if multiple episodes and most recent was Manic Episode; 296.4x if multiple episodes and most recent was Hypomanic Episode.*]

## Bipolar I Disorder: Mixed Episode

[*Interviewer: Code this disorder if criteria are met both for a Manic Episode and for a Major Depressive Episode nearly every day for at least 1 week; disturbance causes clinically significant impairment; and symptoms are not the result of a substance or a general medical condition.*]

☐ Bipolar I Disorder: Mixed Episode (_____)
[*Code 296.6x if most recent episode is mixed; 296.5x if most recent episode is depressed; 296.7 if most recent episode is unspecified.*]

*(cont.)*

## Other Mental and Developmental Disorders

*[Enter 1 if present, 0 if absent, and ? if unknown.]*

1. Does this child have any things about which he/she seems obsessed or can he/she not get his/her mind off of a particular topic? _____ *[If present, review diagnostic criteria for Obsessive–Compulsive Disorder in the DSM-IV.]*
2. Does this child have any unusual behaviors he/she must perform, such as dressing, bathing, mealtime, or counting rituals? _____ *[If present, review diagnostic criteria for Obsessive–Compulsive disorder in the DSM-IV.]*
3. Does this child demonstrate any nervous tics or other repetitive, abrupt nervous movements or vocal noises? _____ *[If present, review diagnostic criteria for Tic Disorders or Tourette's Disorder in the DSM-IV.]*
4. Has this child made comments or acted in such a way that he/she seemed to see things, hear things, or feel things on his/her skin that really did not exist (hallucinations)? _____ *[If present, review diagnostic criteria for Psychotic Disorders in the DSM-IV.]*
5. Has this child ever reported bizarre or very strange or peculiar ideas that seemed very unusual compared to other children (delusions)? _____ *[If present, review diagnostic criteria for Psychotic Disorders in the DSM-IV.]*

### PARENT MANAGEMENT METHODS

Now let's move on and talk about how you have tried to manage your child's behavior, especially when it was a problem for you. When your child is disruptive or misbehaves, what steps are you likely to take to deal with the problem?

_____
_____
_____
_____
_____
_____
_____

If these methods do not work and the problem behavior continues, what are you likely to do then to cope with your child's misbehavior?

_____
_____
_____
_____
_____
_____
_____

*(cont.)*

## CHILD'S EVALUATION AND TREATMENT HISTORY

Has your child ever been evaluated previously for developmental, behavioral, or learning problems? [*Circle one*]    Yes    No

If so, who provided the evaluation, what type of evaluation did the child have, and what were you told about your child regarding the results of any evaluations?

_____

_____

_____

_____

_____

Has your child ever received any psychiatric or psychological treatment? [*Circle one*]   Yes   No

If so, what type of treatment did he/she receive and how long did the treatment last?

_____

_____

Who provided this treatment to your child?_____

Has your child ever received any *medication* for his/her behavior or emotional problems? [*Circle one*]   Yes   No

If so, what type of medication did he/she take, at what dose, and for how long?

_____

_____

## SCHOOL HISTORY

[*Interviewer: For each grade the child has been in, beginning with preschool, ask the parents which school the child attended and whether the child had any behavioral or learning problems that year and, if so, briefly note their nature below.*]

_____

_____

_____

_____

_____

_____

_____

_____

_____

*(cont.)*

Has this child ever received any *special education services*? [*Circle one*]     Yes     No

If so, what types of services did he/she receive and in what grades?

_____

_____

_____

_____

## CHILD'S PSYCHOLOGICAL AND SOCIAL STRENGTHS

I realize I have asked you a lot about any problems your child might be having. But it is also important that I know about your child's psychological and social strong points. Please tell me about any abilities your child seems to have or any activities at which he/she is particularly good. For instance, what hobbies and sports does your child enjoy and do well at, what are his/her best subjects in school, what sorts of games or social activities does he/she do well in? In other words, tell me what you consider to be your child's strongest or best points.

_____

_____

_____

_____

_____

## FAMILY HISTORY

[*Interviewer: After reviewing the child's psychological and social strengths, review with the parent the family history of psychiatric and learning problems, using the following form. One section of the form is for the maternal side of the family, the second for the paternal side, and the third for the siblings of the child being evaluated. Inform the parent(s) you are interviewing that it is important in understanding a child's behavioral problems to know whether other biological relatives of the child have had psychological, emotional, or developmental problems. Many such disorders run in families and may contribute genetically to the child's problems. Start with the maternal side of the family and review each of the mother's relatives, noting whether they have any of the disorders listed on the left side of the form. If so, place an X under the column representing that relative. Then do the same for the paternal relatives and the child's siblings.*]

### Maternal Relatives

| | Self | Mother | Father | Siblings | | | | Total |
|---|---|---|---|---|---|---|---|---|
| | | | | Bro | Bro | Sis | Sis | |
| Problems with aggressiveness, defiance, and oppositional behavior as a child | | | | | | | | |
| Problems with attention, activity, and impulse control as a child | | | | | | | | |

(*cont.*)

| | Self | Mother | Father | Bro | Bro | Sis | Sis | Total |
|---|---|---|---|---|---|---|---|---|
| | | | | \(\) | | Siblings | | |
| Learning disabilities | | | | | | | | |
| Failed to graduate from high school | | | | | | | | |
| Mental retardation | | | | | | | | |
| Psychosis or schizophrenia | | | | | | | | |
| Depression for more than 2 weeks | | | | | | | | |
| Anxiety disorder that impaired adjustment | | | | | | | | |
| Tics or Tourette's | | | | | | | | |
| Alcohol abuse | | | | | | | | |
| Substance abuse | | | | | | | | |
| Antisocial behavior (assaults, thefts, etc.) | | | | | | | | |
| Arrests | | | | | | | | |
| Physical abuse | | | | | | | | |
| Sexual abuse | | | | | | | | |

## Paternal Relatives

| | Self | Mother | Father | Bro | Bro | Sis | Sis | Total |
|---|---|---|---|---|---|---|---|---|
| | | | | | Siblings | | | |
| Problems with aggressiveness, defiance, and oppositional behavior as a child | | | | | | | | |
| Problems with attention, activity, and impulse control as a child | | | | | | | | |
| Learning disabilities | | | | | | | | |
| Failed to graduate from high school | | | | | | | | |
| Mental retardation | | | | | | | | |
| Psychosis or schizophrenia | | | | | | | | |
| Depression for more than 2 weeks | | | | | | | | |
| Anxiety disorder that impaired adjustment | | | | | | | | |
| Tics or Tourette's | | | | | | | | |
| Alcohol abuse | | | | | | | | |
| Substance abuse | | | | | | | | |

(cont.)

| | Self | Mother | Father | Siblings | | | | Total |
|---|---|---|---|---|---|---|---|---|
| | | | | Bro | Bro | Sis | Sis | |
| Antisocial behavior (assaults, thefts, etc.) | | | | | | | | |
| Arrests | | | | | | | | |
| Physical abuse | | | | | | | | |
| Sexual abuse | | | | | | | | |

## Siblings

| | Brother | Brother | Sister | Sister | Total |
|---|---|---|---|---|---|
| Problems with aggressiveness, defiance, and oppositional behavior as a child | | | | | |
| Problems with attention, activity, and impulse control as a child | | | | | |
| Learning disabilities | | | | | |
| Failed to graduate from high school | | | | | |
| Mental retardation | | | | | |
| Psychosis or schizophrenia | | | | | |
| Depression for more than 2 weeks | | | | | |
| Anxiety disorder that impaired adjustment | | | | | |
| Tics or Tourette's | | | | | |
| Alcohol abuse | | | | | |
| Substance abuse | | | | | |
| Antisocial behavior (assaults, thefts, etc.) | | | | | |
| Arrests | | | | | |
| Physical abuse | | | | | |
| Sexual abuse | | | | | |

# ADULT BEHAVIOR RATING SCALE—
# SELF-REPORT OF CURRENT BEHAVIOR (FORM 7)

**Your name** _____ **Age** _____ **Date** _____

**Instructions:** Circle the number that *best describes* your behavior over the past 6 months.

|  | Never or rarely | Sometimes | Often | Very often |
|---|---|---|---|---|
| 1. Fail to give close attention to details or make careless mistakes in job tasks or schoolwork | 0 | 1 | 2 | 3 |
| 2. Have difficulty sustaining attention in tasks or leisure activities | 0 | 1 | 2 | 3 |
| 3. Do not seem to listen when spoken to directly | 0 | 1 | 2 | 3 |
| 4. Do not follow through on instructions and fail to finish work | 0 | 1 | 2 | 3 |
| 5. Have difficulty organizing tasks and activities | 0 | 1 | 2 | 3 |
| 6. Avoid tasks (e.g., job tasks, schoolwork) that require mental effort | 0 | 1 | 2 | 3 |
| 7. Lose things necessary for tasks or activities | 0 | 1 | 2 | 3 |
| 8. Am easily distracted | 0 | 1 | 2 | 3 |
| 9. Am forgetful in daily activities | 0 | 1 | 2 | 3 |
| 10. Fidget with hands or feet or squirm in seat | 0 | 1 | 2 | 3 |
| 11. Leave seat in situations in which remaining seated is expected | 0 | 1 | 2 | 3 |
| 12. Move about excessively in situations in which it is inappropriate; am hyperactive; have feelings of restlessness | 0 | 1 | 2 | 3 |
| 13. Have difficulty engaging in leisure activities quietly | 0 | 1 | 2 | 3 |
| 14. Feel "on the go" or act as if "driven by a motor" | 0 | 1 | 2 | 3 |
| 15. Talk excessively | 0 | 1 | 2 | 3 |
| 16. Blurt out answers before questions have been completed | 0 | 1 | 2 | 3 |
| 17. Have difficulty awaiting turn | 0 | 1 | 2 | 3 |
| 18. Interrupt or intrude on others | 0 | 1 | 2 | 3 |
| 19. Lose temper | 0 | 1 | 2 | 3 |
| 20. Argue with others | 0 | 1 | 2 | 3 |
| 21. Actively defy or refuse to comply with requests or rules | 0 | 1 | 2 | 3 |
| 22. Deliberately annoy people | 0 | 1 | 2 | 3 |
| 23. Blame others for my own mistakes or misbehavior | 0 | 1 | 2 | 3 |
| 24. Am touchy or easily annoyed by others | 0 | 1 | 2 | 3 |
| 25. Feel angry and resentful | 0 | 1 | 2 | 3 |
| 26. Am spiteful or vindictive | 0 | 1 | 2 | 3 |

# ADULT BEHAVIOR RATING SCALE—
## SELF-REPORT OF CHILDHOOD BEHAVIOR (FORM 8)

**Your name** _____ **Age** _____ **Date** _____

**Instructions:** Circle the number that *best describes* your behavior as a child, ages 5–12 years.

| | Never or rarely | Sometimes | Often | Very often |
|---|---|---|---|---|
| 1. Failed to give close attention to details or made careless mistakes in schoolwork | 0 | 1 | 2 | 3 |
| 2. Had difficulty sustaining attention in tasks or play activities | 0 | 1 | 2 | 3 |
| 3. Did not seem to listen when spoken to directly | 0 | 1 | 2 | 3 |
| 4. Did not follow through on instructions and failed to finish work | 0 | 1 | 2 | 3 |
| 5. Had difficulty organizing tasks and activities | 0 | 1 | 2 | 3 |
| 6. Avoided tasks (e.g., schoolwork, homework) that required mental effort | 0 | 1 | 2 | 3 |
| 7. Lost things necessary for tasks or activities | 0 | 1 | 2 | 3 |
| 8. Was easily distracted | 0 | 1 | 2 | 3 |
| 9. Was forgetful in daily activities | 0 | 1 | 2 | 3 |
| 10. Fidgeted with hands or feet or squirmed in seat | 0 | 1 | 2 | 3 |
| 11. Left seat in classroom or in other situations in which remaining seated was expected | 0 | 1 | 2 | 3 |
| 12. Ran about or climbed excessively in situations in which it was inappropriate; was hyperactive | 0 | 1 | 2 | 3 |
| 13. Had difficulty engaging in play activities quietly | 0 | 1 | 2 | 3 |
| 14. Was "on the go" or acted as if "driven by a motor" | 0 | 1 | 2 | 3 |
| 15. Talked excessively | 0 | 1 | 2 | 3 |
| 16. Blurted out answers before questions had been completed | 0 | 1 | 2 | 3 |
| 17. Had difficulty awaiting turn | 0 | 1 | 2 | 3 |
| 18. Interrupted or intruded on others | 0 | 1 | 2 | 3 |
| 19. Lost temper | 0 | 1 | 2 | 3 |
| 20. Argued with adults | 0 | 1 | 2 | 3 |
| 21. Actively defied or refused to comply with requests or rules | 0 | 1 | 2 | 3 |
| 22. Deliberately annoyed people | 0 | 1 | 2 | 3 |
| 23. Blamed others for my own mistakes or misbehavior | 0 | 1 | 2 | 3 |
| 24. Was touchy or easily annoyed by others | 0 | 1 | 2 | 3 |
| 25. Felt angry and resentful | 0 | 1 | 2 | 3 |
| 26. Was spiteful or vindictive | 0 | 1 | 2 | 3 |

# ISSUES CHECKLIST FOR PARENTS AND TEENAGERS (FORM 9)

**Name**_____ **Date**_____

| ☐ Adolescent | | ☐ Adolescent |
|---|---|---|
| ☐ Mother | *with* | ☐ Mother |
| ☐ Father | | ☐ Father |

Below is a list of things that sometimes get talked about at home. We would like you to look carefully at each topic on the left-hand side of the page and decide whether the *two of you together* have talked about that topic at *all* during the last 2 weeks.

If the two of you together have discussed it during the last 2 weeks, circle *Yes* to the right of the topic.

If the two of you together have *not* discussed it during the last 2 weeks, circle No to the right of the topic.

Now, we would like you to go back over the list of topics. For those topics for which you circled Yes, please answer the two questions on the right-hand side of the page.

1. How many times during the last 2 weeks did the topic come up?
2. How hot are the discussions?

Go down this column for all pages first.          Then go down these columns for all pages.

| | | | How many times? | How hot are the discussions? | | | | |
| | | | | Calm | | A little angry | | Angry |
|---|---|---|---|---|---|---|---|---|
| **Topic** | | | | | | | | |
| 1. Telephone calls | Yes | No | | 1 | 2 | 3 | 4 | 5 |
| 2. Time for going to bed | Yes | No | | 1 | 2 | 3 | 4 | 5 |
| 3. Cleaning up bedroom | Yes | No | | 1 | 2 | 3 | 4 | 5 |
| 4. Doing homework | Yes | No | | 1 | 2 | 3 | 4 | 5 |
| 5. Putting away clothes | Yes | No | | 1 | 2 | 3 | 4 | 5 |
| 6. Using the television | Yes | No | | 1 | 2 | 3 | 4 | 5 |

*(cont.)*

| Topic | | | How many times? | Calm | | A little angry | | Angry |
|---|---|---|---|---|---|---|---|---|
| 7. Cleanliness (washing, showers, brushing teeth) | Yes | No | | 1 | 2 | 3 | 4 | 5 |
| 8. Which clothes to wear | Yes | No | | 1 | 2 | 3 | 4 | 5 |
| 9. How neat clothing looks | Yes | No | | 1 | 2 | 3 | 4 | 5 |
| 10. Making too much noise at home | Yes | No | | 1 | 2 | 3 | 4 | 5 |
| 11. Table manners | Yes | No | | 1 | 2 | 3 | 4 | 5 |
| 12. Fighting with brothers or sisters | Yes | No | | 1 | 2 | 3 | 4 | 5 |
| 13. Cursing | Yes | No | | 1 | 2 | 3 | 4 | 5 |
| 14. How money is spent | Yes | No | | 1 | 2 | 3 | 4 | 5 |
| 15. Picking books or movies | Yes | No | | 1 | 2 | 3 | 4 | 5 |
| 16. Allowance | Yes | No | | 1 | 2 | 3 | 4 | 5 |
| 17. Going places without parents (shopping, movies, etc.) | Yes | No | | 1 | 2 | 3 | 4 | 5 |
| 18. Playing stereo or radio too loudly | Yes | No | | 1 | 2 | 3 | 4 | 5 |
| 19. Turning off lights in house | Yes | No | | 1 | 2 | 3 | 4 | 5 |
| 20. Drugs | Yes | No | | 1 | 2 | 3 | 4 | 5 |
| 21. Taking care of records, games, toys, and things | Yes | No | | 1 | 2 | 3 | 4 | 5 |
| 22. Drinking beer or other liquor | Yes | No | | 1 | 2 | 3 | 4 | 5 |
| 23. Buying records, games, toys, and things | Yes | No | | 1 | 2 | 3 | 4 | 5 |
| 24. Going on dates | Yes | No | | 1 | 2 | 3 | 4 | 5 |
| 25. Who should be friends | Yes | No | | 1 | 2 | 3 | 4 | 5 |
| 26. Selecting new clothing | Yes | No | | 1 | 2 | 3 | 4 | 5 |
| 27. Sex | Yes | No | | 1 | 2 | 3 | 4 | 5 |
| 28. Coming home on time | Yes | No | | 1 | 2 | 3 | 4 | 5 |
| 29. Getting to school on time | Yes | No | | 1 | 2 | 3 | 4 | 5 |
| 30. Getting low grades in school | Yes | No | | 1 | 2 | 3 | 4 | 5 |
| 31. Getting in trouble in school | Yes | No | | 1 | 2 | 3 | 4 | 5 |

(cont.)

| Topic | | | How many times? | Calm | | A little angry | | Angry |
|---|---|---|---|---|---|---|---|---|
| 32. Lying | Yes | No | | 1 | 2 | 3 | 4 | 5 |
| 33. Helping out around the house | Yes | No | | 1 | 2 | 3 | 4 | 5 |
| 34. Talking back to parents | Yes | No | | 1 | 2 | 3 | 4 | 5 |
| 35. Getting up in the morning | Yes | No | | 1 | 2 | 3 | 4 | 5 |
| 36. Bothering parents when they want to be left alone | Yes | No | | 1 | 2 | 3 | 4 | 5 |
| 37. Bothering teenager when he/she wants to be left alone | Yes | No | | 1 | 2 | 3 | 4 | 5 |
| 38. Putting feet on furniture | Yes | No | | 1 | 2 | 3 | 4 | 5 |
| 39. Messing up the house | Yes | No | | 1 | 2 | 3 | 4 | 5 |
| 40. What time to have meals | Yes | No | | 1 | 2 | 3 | 4 | 5 |
| 41. How to spend free time | Yes | No | | 1 | 2 | 3 | 4 | 5 |
| 42. Smoking | Yes | No | | 1 | 2 | 3 | 4 | 5 |
| 43. Earning money away from house | Yes | No | | 1 | 2 | 3 | 4 | 5 |
| 44. What teenager eats | Yes | No | | 1 | 2 | 3 | 4 | 5 |

Check to see that you circled "Yes" or "No" for every topic. Then tell the interviewer you are finished.

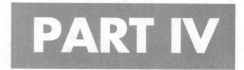

# Family Handouts
# For Steps 1–18

# Contents

*Parent Handout for Step 2: Principles of Behavior Management*     203

*Parent Handout for Step 2: Coercive Behavior Cycle*     204

*Parent Handout for Step 3: Paying Attention to Your Teen's Good Behavior*     205

*Parent Handout for Step 4: How to Give Effective Commands*     207

*Parent Handout for Step 5: Sample Behavioral Contract*     208

*Parent Handout for Step 5: The Home Point System*     210

*Parent Handout for Step 8: Grounding*     211

*Parent Handout for Step 9: Accommodations for Improving Teen School Performance*     212

*Parent Handout for Step 9: 1991 Memorandum from the U.S. Department of Education*     213

*Parent Handout for Step 10: Steps to Better Problem Solving*     219

*Parent Handout for Step 10: Problem-Solving Worksheet*     220

*Parent Handout for Step 10: Problem-Solving Exercise*     221

*Parent Handout for Step 13: Communication Habits*     225

*Parent Handout for Step 15: Unreasonable Beliefs Chart*     226

*Adolescent Handout for Step 15: Unreasonable Beliefs Chart*     230

# PARENT HANDOUT FOR STEP 2: PRINCIPLES OF BEHAVIOR MANAGEMENT

## FOUR-FACTOR MODEL OF TEEN MISBEHAVIOR

Teen factor

Parent factor

Stress

Parenting style

## ABC'S OF BEHAVIORAL MANAGEMENT

Anticipate $\rightarrow$ Behavior $\leftarrow$ Consequences

## REQUESTS AND CONSEQUENCES

| | |
|---|---|
| Specific | Meaningful |
| Immediate | Frequent |
| Consistent | Balanced |

# PARENT HANDOUT FOR STEP 2: COERCIVE BEHAVIOR CYCLE

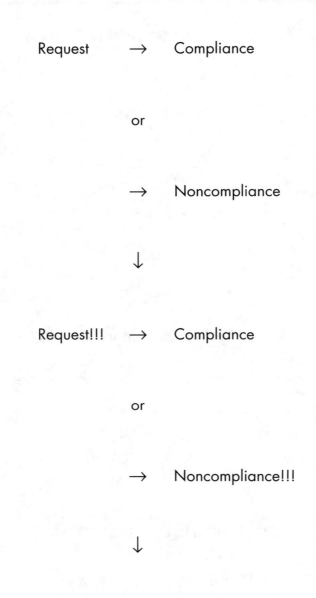

Request    →    Compliance

or

→    Noncompliance

↓

Request!!!  →    Compliance

or

→    Noncompliance!!!

↓

Force or give up

# PARENT HANDOUT FOR STEP 3: PAYING ATTENTION TO YOUR TEEN'S GOOD BEHAVIOR

Like all people, your teenager (let's say a boy) wants to be appreciated for the work he contributes around the home as well as the good behavior he displays to other family members. But, like many of us, he may come to feel taken for granted, that no really appreciates the positive things he contributes to family life or his unique qualities as a person. Although you may feel that your teenager does little that is deserving of appreciation, when you take a more careful look at all of the things he does over the course of a day, you will probably find that not to be true. The purpose of this handout is to help you develop better skills at attending to your teenager's appropriate behavior in hopes that, by doing so, it will increase. When good behavior increases, there is always a corresponding decrease in bad behavior.

Learning to pay attention to the good behavior of others is not an easy thing to do. Many of us do not know how to supervise, manage, or interact with another person so as to increase their desire to work harder for us or follow our rules. Certainly we know how to talk to others, but simply talking to someone may not be very effective at improving our relationship with him/her. It is important to pay attention to *how* we talk to them, *when* we do so, and *what* we say. Effective supervisors have learned skills that make them better able to motivate their employees to work well for them. Like such supervisors, you may need to learn better ways of "supervising" your teenager to improve his motivation to obey and work for you. Here is a list of things which you should try to do to improve your attending skills to your teenager. Your therapist will discuss them in detail with you.

1. Spend at least 15 minutes, three or four times per week, doing something one-on-one with your teen (let's say a girl). The activity should be something enjoyable to the teen, preferably her choice (as long as it is within reason), such as taking a drive to the mall, shooting hoops, playing a video game, and the like. During this limited period of time, **ask no questions, give no directions, make no corrections, give no instructions**. Either make positive comments or neutral descriptive comments. Ignore minor misbehavior. Terminate the activity if the teen becomes disrespectful or violates household rules.

   Alternatively, there will be times when your teen is doing some activity that she enjoys, such as playing a game, building a model, or watching television. Provided her behavior is appropriate, take a minute and go to her to provide some positive attention. When you do this, be sure to be relaxed and casual. Reflect what you think she is doing, such as "It looks like you've got an exciting football game on TV there" or "I see you have started that model car you bought last weekend." Thereafter, look for positive things to say about what the teen is doing, how well she is accomplishing it, or how quiet and well-behaved she is. If you ask questions, do so only for information about what the teen is up to or how she likes what she is doing. Don't ask questions that imply disapproval or criticism, such as "Couldn't you be doing something more useful than watching that boob tube again?" Show interest in what your teen is doing.

   *(cont.)*

2. At times when you are busy and your teen is not bothering you but behaving well, interrupt your activity to go to him and state how much you appreciate his not disturbing you while you work. Done frequently, this will increase the teen's willingness not to disrupt your work when you are busy. Similarly, if he is getting along well with a brother or sister, stop what you are doing to notice it and praise the teen.

3. Whenever your teenager volunteers to help you do something or performs a helpful task around the home without being told, be sure to acknowledge her help and appreciate her effort. It takes only a few seconds to say, "Thanks for helping out with . . ." or "I really appreciate it when you. . . ." Although such things may not seem worthwhile to say, done frequently over time they do produce a significant improvement in your working relationship with your teenager. Don't expect your teenager to show any gratitude for your attention initially, but don't be discouraged. Your teen has heard you and it will have an effect on her behavior.

4. If you ask your teenager to do something, be sure to take a few moments and immediately praise him for beginning to start the task. Giving such positive attention to compliance will eventually increase it.

5. Whenever you are praising or appreciating your teen's behavior, do not use sarcasm or back-handed compliments (for example, "It's about time you cleaned your room"). You may think you are being positive, but you are actually decreasing the odds that she will do this job again for you. Instead, make your statements positive yet accurate. Say precisely what you like about her behavior and even why you like it. Don't exaggerate your praise, as any teen can sense false flattery.

6. The whole secret to being a good supervisor of another person is learning to be attentive to even the small things that others do for us. Be honest, positive, and accurate in your feedback to others. By noticing the little things your teen does for you, may notice a positive change in your relationship with him and an increase in the teen's desire to work for you. If your teenager rejects your initial positive statements with sarcasm, coolness, or disrespect, don't get discouraged. He probably thinks you have an ulterior motive or want something from him. In time, this reaction should pass and he will come to appreciate your attention.

**Remember!! Practice these skills every day as often as you can to improve your relationship with your teen!!**

# PARENT HANDOUT FOR STEP 4: HOW TO GIVE EFFECTIVE COMMANDS

In our work with many behavior-problem teenagers, we have noticed that if parents simply change the way they give commands to their teen, they can often achieve significant improvements in the teen's compliance. When you are about to give a command or instruction to your teen, be sure that you do the following:

1. *Make sure you mean it!* That is, never give a command that you do not intend to see either completed or followed up with a consequence if not completed. When you make a request, plan on backing it up with appropriate consequences, either positive or negative, to show that you mean what you have said.

2. *Do not present the command as a question or favor.* State the command simply, directly, and in a businesslike tone of voice. However, if you truly mean to give the teen a choice, be clear (for example, "Would you like to do your homework now or after supper?" is a legitimate choice; "Would you like to do your homework?" when what is meant is "Do your homework" is not a legitimate choice).

3. *Do not give too many commands at once.* Many teens with ADHD have trouble with multi-step commands. If a task you want your teen to do is complicated, then break it down into smaller steps and give only one step at a time.

4. *Tell the teen what **to do** rather than what **not to do**.* If you state your request in such a way that it provides the teen with information about what his/her next step should be, he/she will be much more likely to comply.

5. *Avoid competing distractions when giving commands.* A very common mistake that parents make is to try to give instructions while a TV, stereo, or video game is on. Parents cannot expect the teen to pay attention to them when something more entertaining is going on in the room. Either turn off these distractions yourself or tell the teen to turn them off before giving the command.

6. *Be cautious of commands that involve the concept of time.* By definition, teens with ADHD experience an impaired perception of time. If parents make requests such as "Have your room cleaned in one hour" or "You have 15 minutes to get ready for school," the teen will probably need some external time marker such as a digital clock a timer set to go off, and the like.

If you follow these six guidelines, you will find some improvement in your teen's compliance with your requests. When used with the other methods your therapist will teach you, significant improvements can occur in how well your teen listens and behaves.

## PARENT HANDOUT FOR STEP 5: SAMPLE BEHAVIORAL CONTRACT

### CONTRACT

This contract between_____(teenager) and

_____(parents) is hereby entered into this, the_____

day of _____, _____.

With regard to _____,

_____(teenager) agrees to:

_____

_____

_____

_____

In return,_____(parents) agree to:

_____

_____

_____

If _____(teenager) does not honor the agreement, the following consequence
is agree upon by both parties:

_____

_____

_____

All parties have read and discussed this agreement. Any exceptions must be mutually agreed upon
by all parties. If disputes arise, changes to the contract may be negotiated in the future.

_____
(Teenager)

_____
(Parents)

_____
(Date)

# PARENT HANDOUT FOR STEP 5: THE HOME POINT SYSTEM

When trying to manage the behavior of a defiant teen, it is common to find that praise is not enough to motivate the teen to do chores, follow rules, or to obey commands. As a result, it is necessary to set up a more powerful program to motivate the teen. One such program that has been very successful with younger teens (ages 12 through 14 or 15 years old) is the home point system. Your therapist will explain in detail how to set up such a program, but here are the steps to follow.

1. Get a notebook, and set it up like a checkbook with five columns, one each for the date, the item, deposits, withdrawals, and the running balance (or actually use a checkbook with only the register portion placed in it). When the teen is rewarded with points, write the job under "item" and enter the amount as a "deposit." Add it to the teen's balance. When the teen "buys" a privilege with his points, note the privilege under "item," place this amount in the withdrawal column, and deduct this amount from the "balance."

2. Make up a list of rewards and privileges. These should include not only occasional special privileges (going to the movies, buying a CD, having a party) but also the every day privileges the teen takes for granted (TV, video games, use of the telephone, etc.). Your therapist will explain what types of privileges you might include on this list. Be sure to have at least 10, half to two thirds of which should be daily privileges.

3. Now make up a second list that will contain the jobs and chores you often ask the teen to perform. These can be typical household chores such as making the bed, washing dishes, putting dirty laundry in the hamper, or emptying the trash. Also put on the list things like getting dressed for school, being in bed by a certain time, getting up for school on time, brushing teeth, or any other self-help task the teen has trouble with. Your therapist can help you decide what types of jobs to put on this list.

4. Next, take each job or chore and decide how much you feel it is worth in points. Use a range of 100 to 1,000 points, and remember, the harder the job, the more points it is worth.

5. Add up approximately how many points you think your teen will earn in a typical day if he/she does most of these jobs. Then, remembering this number, decide how many points your teen should have to pay for each of the privileges you listed. We generally suggest that one half to two thirds of the teen's daily points should be spent on typical daily privileges. This allows the teen to save about one third of his points every day toward the purchase of some of the very special rewards on the list. Don't worry too much about the exact numbers to use here. Just use your judgment as to how much each reward should cost, be fair, and charge more points for the special rewards and less for the daily ones.

6. Be sure to explain the system to the teen before getting started. If the teen expresses resistance, tell him that he will have a chance to earn bonus points when chores are performed in a prompt and pleasant manner. You will not give these bonus points all the time but should give them when your teen has done a job in an especially pleasant and prompt manner.

*(cont.)*

7. Be sure to tell the teen that points will only be given for jobs that are done on the first request. If you have to repeat a command, the teen will not receive any points for doing it.

*Note:* **Do not take points away this week for noncompliance with requests on the list.** After 1 week of earning points, your therapist will explain how to use penalties—points that are deducted when the teen does not comply on the first request or when the teen violates a common household rule.

## OTHER REMINDERS

- Only parents are to write in the point notebook or checkbook register.
- Review the list of privileges and rewards every week or so and add new ones as you deem necessary. Check with your teen for new rewards he/she may want on the list.
- You can reward your teen with bonus points for almost any form of good behavior.
- The teen must have a sufficient number of points in his/her balance in order to purchase a privilege. No credit card mentality!
- Do not give the points before the teen has done what he was told to do, only afterward. Try to do so immediately.

# PARENT HANDOUT FOR STEP 8: GROUNDING

Grounding is the most serious form of punishment used in this program and is reserved for the most significant misbehaviors. Use grounding with only one or two misbehaviors during the first week. Choose those behaviors that are not responding very well to behavioral contracts or the use of penalties.

Warn the teen in advance that if a specific misbehavior occurs, the consequence will be grounding, or "house arrest." This means that for a specified period of time, the teen will have **no access** to anything that the parents define as a privilege.

Grounding must follow the following guidelines:

1. One or both parents must be in the house to enforce the grounding. This may mean that the grounding is postponed until later in the day or later in the week.

2. The period of the "house arrest" lasts anywhere from 2–3 hours to no more than 2 full days. The length of time will depend on the seriousness of the misbehavior as well as the availability of one or both parents to enforce the grounding.

3. During "house arrest," the teen may perform an onerous work detail such as washing windows, sweeping out the basement, and so forth. He will not be paid or rewarded for this job.

4. There may be some items in the house that parents decide are not under their control but truly belong to the teen and which they cannot legitimately withhold from him (for example, a walkman and tapes purchased with the teen's money from a part-time job). This scenario will compromise the effectiveness of grounding and may be justification for using a penalty approach instead.

5. Similarly, an older teen (16, 17, or 18 years old) may have a driver's license and car, and may simply walk out of the house, get into the car, and drive away from grounding. Grounding is not appropriate for teens at this developmental level of maturity, and parents should focus instead on penalties, withholding those valued privileges over which they do have control.

# PARENT HANDOUT FOR STEP 9: ACCOMMODATIONS FOR IMPROVING TEEN SCHOOL PERFORMANCE

- Daily school assignment notebook

- A "case coordinator"

- Extra set of books maintained at home

- Additional school/home tutoring as needed

- Careful scheduling of classes

- Modified homework load

- Oral rather than written demonstration of knowledge

- Large calendars

- Special time and place for homework

- Tape recorder

- Daily/weekly school conduct card (coordinate with point system)

- Untimed tests

- Study hall in the resource room

- Study buddy to contact for missed assignments

- Preferential seating

- Visual teaching tools

- Photocopies of lecture outlines

# PARENT HANDOUT FOR STEP 9: 1991 MEMORANDUM FROM THE U.S. DEPARTMENT OF EDUCATION

**UNITED STATES DEPARTMENT OF EDUCATION**
OFFICE OF SPECIAL EDUCATION AND REHABILITATIVE SERVICES

THE ASSISTANT SECRETARY

MEMORANDUM                    SEP 1 6 1991

DATE        :

TO          :  Chief State School Officers

FROM        :  Robert R. Davila
               Assistant Secretary
               Office of Special Education
                  and Rehabilitative Services

               Michael L. Williams
               Assistant Secretary
               Office for Civil Rights

               John T. MacDonald
               Assistant Secretary
               Office of Elementary
                  and Secondary Education

SUBJECT     :  Clarification of Policy to Address the Needs of
               Children with Attention Deficit Disorders within
               General and/or Special Education

## I.    Introduction

There is a growing awareness in the education community that attention deficit disorder (ADD) and attention deficit hyperactive disorder (ADHD) can result in significant learning problems for children with those conditions. While estimates of the prevalence of ADD vary widely, we believe that three to five percent of school-aged children may have significant educational problems related to this disorder. Because ADD has broad implications for education as a whole, the Department believes it should clarify State and local responsibility under Federal law for addressing the needs of children with ADD in the schools. Ensuring that these students are able to reach their fullest potential is an inherent part of the National education goals and AMERICA 2000. The National goals, and the strategy for achieving them, are based on the assumptions that:   (1) all children can learn and benefit from their education; and (2) the educational community must work to improve the learning opportunities for all children.

---

[1]While we recognize that the disorders ADD and ADHD vary, the term ADD is being used to encompass children with both disorders.

MARYLAND AVE. S.W. WASHINGTON D.C.

---

This memorandum clarifies the circumstances under which children with ADD are eligible for special education services under Part B of the Individuals with Disabilities Education Act (Part B), as well as the Part B requirements for evaluation of such children's unique educational needs. This memorandum will also clarify the responsibility of State and local educational agencies (SEAs and LEAs) to provide special education and related services to eligible children with ADD under Part B. Finally, this memorandum clarifies the responsibilities of LEAs to provide regular or special education and related aids and services to those children with ADD who are not eligible under Part B, but who fall within the definition of "handicapped person" under Section 504 of the Rehabilitation Act of 1973. Because of the overall educational responsibility to provide services for these children, it is important that general and special education coordinatetheir efforts.

II.     Eligibility for Special Education and Related Services under Part B

Last year during the reauthorization of the Education of the Handicapped Act (now the Individuals with Disabilities Education Act), Congress gave serious consideration to including ADD in the definition of "children with disabilities" in the statute. The Department took the position that ADD does not need to be added as a separate disability category in the statutory definition since children with ADD who require special education and related services can meet the eligibility criteria for services under Part B. This continues to be the Department's position.

No change with respect to ADD was made by Congress in the statutory definition of "children with disabilities;" however, language was included in Section 102(a) of the Education of the Handicapped Act Amendments of 1990 that required the Secretary to issue a Notice of Inquiry (NOI) soliciting public comment on special education for children with ADD under Part B. In response to the NOI (published November 29, 1990 in the Federal Register), the Department received over 2000 written comments, which have been transmitted to the Congress. Our review of these written comments indicates that there is confusion in the field regarding the extent to which children with ADD may be served in special education programs conducted under Part B.

A.     Description of Part B

Part B requires SEAs and LEAs to make a free appropriate public education (FAPE) available to all eligible children with disabilities and to ensure that the rights and protections of Part B are extended to those children and their parents 20 U.S.C. 1412(2); 34 CFR SS300.121 and 300.2. Under Part B, FAPE, among other elements, includes the provision of special education and related services, at no cost to parents, in conformity with an individualized education program (IEP). 34 CFR §300.4.

In order to be eligible under Part B, a child must be evaluated in accordance with 34 CFR §§300.530-300.534 as having one or more specified physical or mental impairments, and must be found to require special education and related services by reason of one or more of these impairments.[2] 20 U.S.C. 1401 (a) (1); 34 CFR §300.5. SEAs and LEAs must ensure that children with ADD who are determined eligible for services under Part B receive special education and related services designed to meet their unique needs, including special education and related services needs arising from the ADD. A full continuum of placement alternatives, including the regular classroom, must be available for providing special education and related services required in the IEP.

B.     Eligibility for Part B services under the "Other Health Impaired" Category

The list of chronic or acute health problems included within the definition of "other health impaired" in the Part B regulations is not exhaustive. The term "other health impaired" includes chronic or acute impairments that result in limited alertness, which

---

[2]The Part B regulations define 11 specified disabilities. 34 CFR §300.5(b) (1)-(11). The Education of the Handicapped Act Amendments of 1990 amended the Individuals with Disabilities Education Act (formerly the Education of the Handicapped Act) to specify that autism and traumatic brain injury are separate disability categories. See section 602(a) (1) of the Act, to be codified at 20 U.S.C. 1401(a) (1).

adversely affects educational performanc. Thus, children with ADD should be classified as eligible for services under the "other health impaired" category in instances where the ADD is a chronic or acute health problem that results in limited alertness. which adversely affects educational performance. In other words, children with ADD, where the ADD is a chronic or acute health problem resulting in limited alertness, may be considered disabled under Part B solely on the basis of this disorder within the "other health impaired" category in situations where special education and related services are needed because of the ADD.

C.    Eligibility for Part B services under Other Disability Categories

Children with ADD are also eligible for services under Part B if the children satisfy the criteria applicable to other disability categories. For example, children with ADD are also eligible for services under the "specific learning disability" category of Part B if they meet the criteria stated in §§300.5(b) (9) and 300.541 or under the "seriously emotionally disturbed" category of Part B if they meet the criteria stated i §300.5(b) (8).

III.    Evaluations under Part B

A.    Requirements

SEAs and LEAs have an affirmative obligation to evaluate a child who is suspected of having a disability to determine the child's need for special education and related services. Under Part B, SEA's and LEAs are required to have procedures for locating, identifying and evaluating all children who have a disability or are suspected of having a disability and are in need of special education and related services. 34 CFR §§300.128 and 300.220. This responsibility, known as "child find," is applicable to all children from birth through 21, regardless of the severity of their disability.

Consistent with this responsibility and the obligation to make FAPE available to all eligible children with disabilities, SEAs and LEAs must ensure that evaluations of children who are suspected of needing special education and related services are conducted without undue delay. 20 U.S.C. 1412(2). Because of its responsibility resulting from the FAPE and child find requirements of Part B, an LEA may not refuse to evaluate the possible need for special education and related services of a child with a prior medical diagnosis of ADD solely by reason of that medical diagnosis. However, a medical diagnosis of ADD alone is not sufficient to render a child eligible for services under Part B.

Under Part B, before any action is taken with respect to the initial placement of a child with a disability in a program providing special education and related services, "a full and individual evaluation of the child's educational needs must be conducted in accordance with requirements of §300.532." 34  CFR §300.531. Section 300.532(a) requires that a child's evaluation must be conducted by a multidisciplinary team, including at least one teacher or other specialist with knowledge in the area of suspected disability.

B.    Disagreements over Evaluations

Any proposal or refusal of an agency to initiate or change the identification, evaluation, or educational placement of the child, or the provision of FAPE to the child is subject to the written prior notice requirements of 34 CFR §§300.504-300.505.[3] If a parent

---

[3]Section 300.505 of the Part B regulations sets out the elements that must be contained in the prior written notice to parents:

(1) A full explanation of all of the procedural safeguards available to the parents under Subpart E;
(2) A description of the action proposed or refused by the agency, an explanation of why the agency proposes or refuses to take the action, and a description of any options the agency considered and the reasons why those options were rejected;

disagrees with the LEA's refusal to evaluate a child or the LEA's evaluation and determination that a child does not have a disability for which the child is eligible for services under Part B, the parent may request a due process hearing pursuant to 34 CFR §§300.506-300.513 of the Part B regulations.

IV.    Obligations Under Section 504 of SEAs and LEAs to Children with ADD Found Not To Require Special Education and Related Services under Part B

Even if a child with ADD is found not to be eligible for services under Part B, the requirements of Section 504 of the Rehabilitation Act of 1973 (Section 504) and its implementing regulation at 34 CFR Part 104 may be applicable. Section 504 prohibits discrimination on the basis of handicap by recipients of Federal funds. Since Section 504 is a civil rights law, rather than a funding law, its requirements are framed in different terms than those of Part B. While the Section 504 regulation was written with an eye to consistency with Part B, it is more general, and there are some differences arising from the differing natures of the two laws. For instance, the protections of Section 504 extend to some children who do not fall within the disability categories specified in Part B.

A.    Definition

Section 504 requires every recipient that operates a public elementary or secondary education program to address the needs of children who are considered "handicapped persons" under Section 504 as adequately as the needs of nonhandicapped persons are met. "Handicapped person" is defined in the Section 504 regulation as any person who has a physical or mental impairment which substantially limits a major life activity (e.g., learning). 34 CFR §104.3(j). Thus, depending on the severity of their condition, children with ADD may fit within that definition.

B.    Programs and Services Under Section 504

Under Section 504, an LEA must provide a free appropriate public education to each qualified handicapped child. A free appropriate public education, under Section 504, consists of regular or special education and related aids and services that are designed to meet the individual student's needs and based on adherence to the regulator requirements on educational setting, evaluation, placement, and procedural safeguards. 34 CFR §§104.33, 104.34, 104.35, and 104.36. A student may be handicapped within the meaning of Section 504, and therefore entitled to regular or special education and related aids and services under the Section 504 regulation, even though the student may not be eligible for special education and related services under Part B.

Under Section 504, if parents believe that their child is handicapped by ADD, the LEA must evaluate the child to determine whether he or she is handicapped as defined by Section 504. If an LEA determines that a child is not handicapped under Section 504, the parent has the right to contest that determination. If the child is determined to be handicapped under Section 504, the LEA must make an individualized determination of the child's educational needs for regular or special education or related aids and services. 34 CFR §104.35. For children determined to be handicapped under Section 504, implementation of an individualized education program developed in accordance with Part B, although not required, is one means of meeting the free appropriate public education requirements of Section 504.[4] The child's education must be provided in the

---

(3) A description of each evaluation procedure, test, record, or report the agency uses as a basis for the proposal or refusal; and
(4) A description of any other factors which are relevant to the agency's proposal or refusal.

    [4]Many LEAs use the same process for determining the needs of students under Section 504 that they use for implementing Part B.

regular education classroom unless it is demonstrated that education in the regular environment with the use of supplementary aids and services cannot be achieved satisfactorily. 34 CFR §104.34.

Should it be determined that the child with ADD is handicapped for purposes of Section 504 and needs only adjustments in the regular classroom, rather than special education, those adjustments are required by Section 504. A range of strategies is available to meet the educational needs of children with ADD. Regular classroom teachers are important in identifying the appropriate educational adaptions and interventions for many children with ADD.

SEAs and LEAs should take the necessary steps to promote coordination between special and regular education programs. Steps also should be taken to train regular education teachers and other personnel to develop their awareness about ADD and its manifestations and the adaptations that can be implemented in regular education programs to address the instructional needs of these children. Examples of adaptations in regular education programs could include the following:

> providing a structured learning environment; repeating and simplifying instructions about in-class and homework assignments; supplementing verbal instructions with visual instructions; using behavioral management techniques; adjusting class schedules; modifying test delivery; using tape recorders, computer-aided instrction, and other audiovisual equipment; selecting modified textbooks or workbooks; and tailoring homework assignments.

Other provisions range from consultation to special resources and may include reducing class size; use of one-on-one tutorials; classroom aides and note takers; involvement of a "services coordinator" to oversee implementation of special programs and services, and possible modification of nonacademic times such as lunchroom, recess, and physical education.

Through the use of appropriate adaptations and interventions in regular classes, many of which may be required by Section 504, the Department believes that LEAs will be able to effectively address the instructional needs of many children with ADD.

C.    Procedural Safeguards Under Section 504

Procedural safeguards under the Section 504 regulation are stated more generally than in Part B. The Section 504 regulation requires the LEA to make available a system of procedural safeguards that permits parents to challenge actions regarding the identification, evaluation, or educational placement of their handicapped child whom they believe needs special education or related services. 34 CFR §104.36. The Section 504 regulation requires that the system of procedural safeguards include notice, an opportunity for the parents or guardian to examine relevant records, an impartial hearing with opportunity for participation by the parents or guardian and representation by counsel, and a review procedure. Compliance with procedural safeguards of Part B is one means of fulfilling the Section 504 requirements.[5] However, in an impartial due process hearing raising issues under the Section 504 regulation, the impartial hearing officer must make a determination based upon that regulation.

V.    Conclusion

Congress and the Department have recognized the need to provide information and assistance to teachers, administrators, parents and other interested persons regarding the identification, evaluation, and instructional needs of children with ADD. The Department has formed a work group to explore strategies across principal offices to address this issue. The work group also plans to identify some ways that the Department

---

[5] Again, many LEAs and some SEAs are conserving time and resources by using the same due process procedures for resolving disputes under both laws.

can work with the education associations to cooperatively consider the programs and services needed by children with ADD across special and regular education.

In fiscal year 1991, the Congress appropriated funds for the Department to synthesize and disseminate current knowledge related to ADD. Four centers will be established in Fall, 1991 to analyze and synthesize the current research literature on ADD relating to identification, assessment, and interventions. Research syntheses will be prepared in formats suitable for educators, parents and researchers. Existing clearinghouses and networks, as well as Federal, State and local organizations will be utilized to disseminate these research syntheses to parents, educators and administrators, and other interested persons.

In addition, the Federal Resource Center will work with SEAs and the six regional resource centers authorized under the Individuals with Disabilities Education Act to identfy effective identification and assessment procedures, as well as intervention strategies being implemented across the country for children with ADD. A document describing current practice will be developed and disseminated to parents, educators and administrators, and other interested persons through the regional resource centers, network, as well as by parent training centers, other parent and consumer organizations, and professional organizations. Also, the Office for Civil Rights' ten regional offices stand ready to provide technical assistance to parents and educators.

It is our hope that the above information will be of assistance to your State as you plan for the needs of children with ADD who require special education and related services under Part B, as well as for the needs of the broader group of children with ADD who do not qualify for special education and related services under Part B, but for whom special education or adaptations in regular education programs are needed. If you have any questions, please contact Jean Peelen, Office for Civil Rights; (Phone: 202/732-1635), Judy Schrag, Office of Special Education Programs (Phone: 202/732-1007); or Dan Bonner, Office of Elementary and Secondary Education (Phone: 202/401-0984).

# PARENT HANDOUT FOR STEP 10: STEPS TO BETTER PROBLEM SOLVING

1. Define the problem—then stick to it

↓

2. Brain storm: Think of as many possible solutions as you can

↓

3. Evaluate your options

↓

4. Select the option most agreeable to all

↓

5. Implement the plan

↓

6. Evaluate the implementation of the plan

- Go back to Step 2 if necessary

- Go back to Step 1 if necessary

- Establish consequences if necessary

# PARENT HANDOUT FOR STEP 10: PROBLEM-SOLVING WORKSHEET

Date_____

Problem_____

_____

|  | Evaluations | | |
| Proposed solutions | Teen<br>+ − | Mother<br>+ − | Father<br>+ − |
| 1._____ | | | |
| 2._____ | | | |
| 3._____ | | | |
| 4._____ | | | |
| 5._____ | | | |
| 6._____ | | | |
| 7._____ | | | |
| 8._____ | | | |
| 9._____ | | | |
| 10._____ | | | |
| 11._____ | | | |
| 12._____ | | | |

Agreement_____

## IMPLEMENTATION PLAN

A. Teen will do:_____ by the following
   time: _____.

B. Mom will do:_____ by the
   following time: _____.

C. Dad will do:_____ by the following
   time: _____.

D. Plan for monitoring whether this happens: _____
_____

E. Any reminders that will be given. By whom? When? _____

F. Consequences for compliance and noncompliance:_____
_____

# PARENT HANDOUT FOR STEP 10: PROBLEM-SOLVING EXERCISE

Name _____ Date _____

The purpose of this worksheet is to give you practice with the steps of problem solving. Write out the answers as best you can. Bring the sheet to your therapist at your next session; the therapist will go over it with you.

## I. Defining the problem
A good definition of the problem explains what it is that the other person is doing or saying that bothers you and why it bothers you. The definition is short, neutral, and does not blame the other person. Below are several definitions. Read each one, then say whether it is good or bad. If it is bad, write down a better definition.

A. **Mother:**  My problem is that I don't like to see your room dirty; all the clothes are on the bed and the dust is two inches thick. I'm upset when my friends come to visit and see the room looking that way.

    1. Is this a good definition of a room-cleaning problem?
         _____ Yes _____ No

    2. If you said No, write a better definition: _____

    _____

    _____

    _____

B. **Daughter:** I hate you, Mom. You just are a real pain. I'm missing out on all the fun because you make me come home by 9 P.M. on weekends.

    1. Is this a good definition of a coming-home-on-time problem?
         _____ Yes _____ No

    2. If you said No, write a better definition: _____

    _____

    _____

    _____

C. **Father:**  Son, the real problem with you is that you don't respect your elders. Kids just don't know the meaning of respect today. When I was your age I would never talk to my father the way you talk to me.

    1. Is this a good definition of a talking-back problem?
         _____ Yes _____ No

*(cont.)*

2. If you said No, write a better definition:_____

_____

_____

_____

D. **Son:** I get angry when you bug me 10 times a day about taking out the trash and feeding the dogs. I'm old enough to do these things without being reminded.

    1. Is this a good definition of a chores problem?

    _____ Yes   _____ No

    2. If you said No, write a better definition:_____

_____

_____

_____

E. Below, a mother and a daughter define their problem about playing the stereo too loud. Notice how each accuses and blames the other; this is a poor way to define the problem. Read their definitions, then write a better definition for each person.

**Mother:** You are ruining your ears with that loud stereo. You just don't have good taste in music. How can you stand all that loud noise? I can't, and what's more, I *won't* stand for it.

**Daughter:** Don't talk to me about taste in music. You sit around all day listening to 1940 junk music. No one listens to that stuff anymore. And get off my back about the loud stereo. I'll play it as loud as I like so I can enjoy my music.

Better definitions:

    **Mother:** _____

_____

_____

_____

    **Daughter:** _____

_____

_____

_____

## II. Listing solutions

A. List as many ideas as you can.
B. Be creative and free.
C. Anything goes.
D. Don't say whether ideas are good or bad now—this comes later. Make believe you are trying to solve a telephone problem: A mother is upset because her son talks on the phone 2 hours a night and runs up bills. The son says his friends live too far away to visit on week-

(cont.)

days; he calls them instead. Make a list of 10 ideas to solve this problem. Put down anything you can think of. Try to be creative.

List of solutions:

1. _____

2. _____

3. _____

4. _____

5. _____

6. _____

7. _____

8. _____

9. _____

10. _____

If you run out of ideas, here are some hints:

- Is a trade-off possible?
- Can they change anything around the house to help?
- Is a change of place or time possible?
- What about other ways to talk to friends?

## III. Picking the best idea: decision making

When you decide on the best idea, you should state the good and bad points of each idea on you list. Then rate each idea "+" or "–". Ask yourself about each idea:

A. Will this idea solve my problem?
B. Will this idea solve the other person's problem?
C. Will this idea really work?
D. Can I live with it?

Consider the telephone problem we discussed above. Make believe one idea was "buy a second telephone."

1. An adolescent might evaluate this as follows: "Well, this idea meets my need to talk to my friends, and my mother might get off my back for talking on her phone too much. I'll give it a '+'."

2. A parent might evaluate it as follows: "It is true that this would get my son off my phone, but it would not solve the problem of high bills—we would have to pay for two phones. Now, if my son wants to get a job to pay for the new phone, that's different. As is, I rate this idea '–'."

(cont.)

Now write out evaluations of the first two solutions to the telephone problem from your list on the last page. For each idea write out an evaluation from the parent's side and a second evaluation from the adolescent's side.

**Idea 1**

Parent's evaluation: _____

_____

_____

_____

Adolescent's evaluation: _____

_____

_____

_____

**Idea 2**

Parent's evaluation: _____

_____

_____

Adolescent's evaluation: _____

_____

_____

_____

# PARENT HANDOUT FOR STEP 13: COMMUNICATION HABITS

| Poor | Good |
| --- | --- |
| Insults | State the issue |
| Interrupts | Take turns |
| Criticizes | Note good and bad |
| Gets defensive | Calmly disagree |
| Lectures | Short and straight |
| Looks away | Make eye contact |
| Slouches | Sit up straight |
| Sarcasm | Talk in normal tone |
| Goes silent | Say what you feel |
| Denial | Accept responsibility |
| Commands, orders | Ask nicely |
| Yells | Use normal tone of voice |
| Swears | Use emphatic but respectful language |
| Throws a tantrum | Cool it, count to 10, take a hike |

## GENERAL PRINCIPLES OF GOOD COMMUNICATION

1. Listen when your teen/parent is in the mood to talk, but don't force him/her to open up.
2. Use active listening to encourage your teen/parent to express opinions and feelings.
3. Honestly express how you feel, good or bad, without being hurtful to your listeners.

# PARENT HANDOUT FOR STEP 15: UNREASONABLE BELIEFS CHART

## PARENTS

Perfectionism/obedience

Ruination

Malicious intent

Appreciation/indulgence

## ADOLESCENT

Unfairness/ruination

Autonomy

Love/appreciation

| Unreasonable beliefs | Reasonable beliefs |
|---|---|
| I. **Perfection/obedience:** Teens with ADHD should behave perfectly and obey their parents all of the time without question. | I. It is unrealistic to expect teens with ADHD to behave perfectly or obey all of the time; we strive for high standards but accept imperfections. |
| A. School<br>1. He should always compete homework on time. | 1. I will encourage him to complete homework all the time but will recognize this won't always happen. |
| 2. She should study 2 hours every night, even when she has no homework. | 2. If your attention span is short, you are lucky to get basic homework done. Extra study is just unrealistic. These kids need a break after all the effort it takes to do basic homework. |
| 3. He should always come to class prepared. | 3. He will sometimes come to class unprepared, but I will help him learn good organizational techniques. |
| 4. She should do papers for the love of learning. | 4. Research shows teens with ADHD need salient, external reinforcers to motivate their behavior. *C'est la vie.* |
| B. Driving<br>1. He should never get any speeding tickets. | 1. All teens with ADHD get at least one speeding ticket. He should be responsible for paying it and take his medicine while driving. |
| 2. She will never have an accident. | 2. Research shows most teens with ADHD will get in at least one minor accident. She should take her medicine when she will be driving, and do her best. She should drive an old car. |
| 3. Teens shouldn't adjust the radio tuner while driving down the highway. | 3. He should avoid tuning the radio while driving as much as possible, but this may occasionally happen. |
| 4. She will always stop completely for stop signs. | 4. I should stop completely at stop signs to model good behavior when my teen is in my car. I can only expect my teen to do as well as I do. |
| C. Conduct<br>1. He should be a perfect angel in church. | 1. This is unrealistic. As long as there are no major disturbances, I'm satisfied. Perhaps I should find a youth group service of more interest for him anyway. |

*(cont.)*

| Unreasonable beliefs | Reasonable beliefs |
|---|---|
| 2. She will impress all the relatives with her love for family gatherings. | 2. Give her space. Teens just don't want to be with their families that much. This is normal. She should attend some family functions, but that is all I can reasonably expect. |
| 3. He should never treat us disrespectfully. | 3. You can't become your own person without some rebellion. Some back-talk is natural. He shouldn't curse or ridicule severely, and might be expected to apologize occasionally. |
| 4. She should get out of a bad mood when we tell her to change her attitude. | 4. People with ADHD are just moody and can't stop it. She should let us know when she is in a bad mood and keep to herself. We should not make a lot of demands on her at such times. |

D. Chores

| | |
|---|---|
| 1. She should put away the dishes the first time I ask. | 1. It won't always happen the first time, but after several reminders, I should act, not yak: apply consequences. |
| 2. He should always get the room spotless. | 2. He should get it generally neat. Spotless isn't realistic. |
| 3. She should not waste electricity by leaving the lights on. | 3. She is just forgetful. We could work out a reminder system, but this is the least of my worries with a teen with ADHD. |
| 4. He shouldn't be on the telephone when I've sent him to clean up his room. | 4. Teens with ADHD will get off task; I will redirect him back to the task, and if it happens too much, assume it is defiance and ground him from the telephone. |

| | |
|---|---|
| II. **Ruination:** If I give my teen too much freedom, she will mess up, make bad judgments, get into big trouble, and ruin his/her life. | II. She will sometimes mess up with too much freedom, but this is how teenagers learn responsibility—a bit of freedom and a bit of responsibility. If she backslides, no big deal. I just pull back on the freedom for a while, and then give her another chance. |
| A. Room incompletely cleaned: he will grow up to be a slovenly, unemployed, aimless welfare case. | A. The state of his room has little to do with how he turns out when he grows up. |

*(cont.)*

| Unreasonable beliefs | Reasonable beliefs |
|---|---|
| B. Home late: she will have unprotected sex, get pregnant, dump the baby on us, take drugs, and drink alcohol. | B. I have no evidence that she would do all these things. She is just self-centered and focused on having fun. So she will be punished as we agreed for coming home late. |
| C. Fighting with siblings: He will never learn to get along with others, have friends, have close relationships, or get married. He will end up a loser and be severely depressed or commit suicide. | C. There is no scientific evidence that sibling fighting predicts later satisfaction in relationships. Siblings always fight. They will probably be closer when they grow up. |
| III. **Malicious intent:** My son misbehaves on purpose to annoy me or to get even with me for restricting him. | III. Most of the time adolescents with ADHD just do things without thinking. They aren't planful enough to connive to upset parents on purpose. |
| A. Talking disrespectfully: She mouths off on purpose to get even with me for_____. | A. Impulsive teenagers just mouth off when frustrated. I'll try not to take it to heart. |
| B. Doesn't follow directions: He purposefully doesn't finish mowing the grass just to get me angry. | B. Teens with ADHD are allergic to effort. They don't take the time to plan to upset parents by not doing things. |
| C. Restless behavior: She shuffles her feet and plays with her hair to get on my nerves. | C. Teens with ADHD just can't contain themselves. I'll try not to attach meaning to her restlessness and ignore it. |
| D. Spending money impulsively: He He bought $100 of CDs just to waste our money. | D. He probably just saw the CDs and had to have them. Poor delay of gratification is part of ADHD. She won't get any extra money for lunch or gas. |
| IV. **Appreciation/indulgence:** My teen should appreciate all of the great sacrifices I make. Showing indulgence or buying things for my teenager is the best way to show love. | IV. Teens with ADHD are so self-centered they don't easily show appreciation until they grow up and have their own children with ADHD. Indulgence reinforces coercion; it doesn't teach responsibility. |
| A. Money: What does he mean he wants more allowance? He should be grateful for all the money I spend on him now. Some kids are not so lucky. | A. He will have to earn more allowance. I'd appreciate a thank you even though I understand he doesn't really think about what I do for him. |
| B. Gifts: If I give her a large gift, she will then appreciate me and do what I say. | B. If I give her a large gift, she may expect large gifts all the time and become spoiled and manipulative. |
| C. Unconditional love: She needs to be loved and accepted no matter what she does or how she act. | C. Unconditional acceptance is important, but I don't want to reinforce bad behavior. |

# ADOLESCENT HANDOUT FOR STEP 15:
# UNREASONABLE AND REASONABLE BELIEFS

| Unreasonable beliefs | Reasonable beliefs |
|---|---|
| I. **Unfairness/ruination:** My parents' rules are totally unfair. I'll never have a good time or any friends. My parents are ruining my life with their unfair rules. They just don't understand me. | I. Yes, I don't like my parents rules and maybe they are sometimes unfair. But who said life is supposed to be fair? And how many other teenagers have gone through the same thing? They turned out OK. So will I. I'll just have to put up with it the best I can. |
| A. Curfew: Why should I have to come home earlier than my friends? They will think I'm a baby. I'll lose all my friends. | A. My friends are loyal. They will understand that my parents are creeps about curfew. I won't lose any friends. |
| B. Chores: Why do I get stuck doing all of the work? My brother doesn't have to do anything. That's unfair! | B. My brother has some chores too. I'll count them up and if I have more, I'll talk nicely to my parents about it. |
| C. School: My teacher is unfair. She picks on me all the time. I always get stuck doing extra homework. I'll never have time for fun. Life is one big homework assignment. | C. Maybe she does pick on me. There could be a reason. I never am with the class or know the answer when she calls on me. Maybe if I kept up with the work she wouldn't call on me so much. |
| II. **Autonomy:** I ought to have complete and total freedom. My parents shouldn't boss me around or tell me what to do. I'm old enough for freedom now. | II. No teen has complete freedom. No adult really does either. Sometimes I need my parents, like for money or God forbid, even to talk to in times of trouble. I want a lot of freedom, but not total freedom. |
| A. Chores: I don't need any reminders. I can do it totally on my own. | A. I have not been getting them done on my own. I need to stop being an asshole and accept a little help. |
| B. Medicine: I don't need Ritalin anymore. I'm grown up now and can handle everything on my own. | B. Maybe I need to see whether I do better or worse on or off medicine. I'll keep an open mind about it. |
| C. Smoking: It's my body. I can do whatever I want with it. You have no right to tell me not to smoke. | C. It's my body. But do I really want to mess it up? My friends have gotten hookedon smoking. It costs a lot. And it tastes terrible when you kiss. |

(cont.)

---

III. **Love/appreciation:** Getting material things is a sign that your parents love you. Getting your way is a sign that your parents really love you.

    A. Clothes: If my parents really loved me, they would let me buy those designer clothes.

    B. Concert: If my parents really loved me, they would let me go to the rock concert with my friends.

    C. Sexuality: If I have sex with my boyfriend, then he will really love me forever and marry me.

III. Material things don't tell you whether someone really cares about you. Sex doesn't make people really care about you either. It's how you are inside that makes the difference.

    A. I would like designer clothes but that's not how I tell whether my parents love me. I can tell from how they act towards me and the affection they show.

    B. If they really love me and think it is dangerous to go to the concert, they are going to try to stop me. I won't use this to judge how they feel.

    C. Love does not equal sex. I need to judge from how my boyfriend acts and expresses his feelings to me whether he loves me. All boys want sex. So this tells me nothing about love.

# References

Abidin, R. R. (1986). *The Parenting Stress Index*. Charlottesville, VA: Pediatric Psychology Press.

Abikoff, H., & Hechtman, L. (1995, June). *Preliminary results of a multi-modal treatment program for ADHD children*. Paper presented at the annual meeting of the International Society for Research in Child and Adolescent Psychopathology, London.

Achenbach, T. M. (1991). *Child Behavior Checklist—Cross-Informant Version*. Burlington, VT: Author.

Achenbach, T. M., & Edelbrock, C. (1983). *Manual for the Child Behavior Checklist and Revised Child Behavior Profile*. Burlington, VT: Thomas Achenbach.

Achenbach, T. M., & Edelbrock, C. (1986). *Manual for the Teacher Report Form and the Child Behavior Profile*. Burlington, VT: Thomas Achenbach.

Achenbach, T. M., & Edelbrock, C. (1987). *Manual for the Child Behavior Checklist Youth Self Report*. Burlington, VT: Thomas Achenbach.

Achenbach, T. M., McConaughy, S. H., & Howell, C. T. (1987). Child/adolescent behavioral and emotional problems: Implications of cross-informant correlations for situational specificity. *Psychological Bulletin, 101*, 213–232.

Adams, C. D., McCarthy, M., & Kelley, M. L. (1995). Adolescent versions of the Home and School Situations Questionnaires: Initial psychometric properties. *Journal of Child Clinical Psychology, 24*, 377–385.

Altepeter, T. S., & Breen, M. J. (1992). Situational variation in problem behavior at home and school in attention deficit disorder with hyperactivity: A factor analytic study. *Journal of Child Psychology and Psychiatry, 33*, 741–748.

American Psychiatric Association (APA). (1980). *Diagnostic and statistical manual of mental disorders* (3rd ed.). Washington, DC: Author.

American Psychiatric Association (APA). (1987). *Diagnostic and statistical manual of mental disorders* (3rd ed., rev.). Washington, DC: Author.

American Psychiatric Association (APA). (1994). *Diagnostic and statistical manual of mental disorders* (4th ed.). Washington, DC: Author.

Anastopoulos, A. D., Guevremont, D. C., Shelton, T. L., & DuPaul, G. J. (1992). Parenting stress among families of children with attention deficit hyperactivity disorder. *Journal of Abnormal Child Psychology, 20*, 503–520.

Anastopoulos, A. D., Shelton, T. L., DuPaul, G. J., & Guevremont, D. C. (1993). Parent training for attention-deficit hyperactivity disorder: Its impact on parent functioning. *Journal of Abnormal Child Psychology, 21*, 581–596.

Applegate, B., Lahey, B. B., Hart, E. L., Waldman, I., Biederman, J., Hynd, G. W., Barkley, R. A., Ollendick, T., Frick, P. J., Greenhill, L., McBurnett, K., Newcorn, J., Kerdyk, L., Garfinkel, B., & Shaffer, D. (1997). The age of onset for DSM-IV attention-deficit hyperactivity disorder: A report of the DSM-IV field trials. *Journal of the American Academy of Child and Adolescent Psychiatry, 36*, 1211–1221.

Asher, S. R., & Coie, J. D. (1990). *Peer rejection in childhood*. New York: Cambridge University Press.

Atkeson, B. M., & Forehand, R. (1978). Parent behavioral training for problem children: An examination of studies using multiple outcome measures. *Journal of Abnormal Child Psychology, 6*, 449–460.

Barkley, R. A. (1981). *Hyperactive children: A handbook for diagnosis and treatment*. New York: Guilford Press.

Barkley, R. A. (1985). The social interactions of hyperactive children: Developmental changes, drug effects, and situational variation. In R. McMahon & R. Peters (Eds.), *Childhood disorders: Behavioral–developmental approaches* (pp. 218–243). New York: Brunner/Mazel.

Barkley, R. A. (1987). *Defiant children: A clinician's manual for parent training*. New York: Guilford Press.

Barkley, R. A. (1988). Child behavior rating scales and checklists. In M. Rutter, A. H. Tuma, & I. S. Lann (Eds.), *Assessment and diagnosis in child psychopathology* (pp. 113–155). New York: Guilford Press.

Barkley, R. A. (1990). *Attention deficit hyperactivity disorder: A handbook for diagnosis and treatment*. New York: Guilford Press.

Barkley, R. A. (1992a). *ADHD: What do we know?* (Videotape). New York: Guilford Press.

Barkley, R. A. (1992b). *ADHD: What can we do?* (Videotape). New York: Guilford Press.

Barkley, R. A. (1996). Attention-deficit/hyperactivity disorder. In E. J. Mash & R. A. Barkley (Eds.), *Child psychopathology* (pp. 63–112). New York: Guilford Press.

Barkley, R. A. (1997a). Behavioral inhibition, sustained attention, and executive functions: Constructing a unifying theory of ADHD. *Psychological Bulletin, 121*, 64–95.

Barkley, R. A. (1997b). *Defiant children* (2nd ed.): *A clinician's manual for assessment and parent training*. New York: Guilford Press.

Barkley, R. A. (1997c). *Managing the defiant child* (Videotape). New York: Guilford Press.

Barkley, R. A. (1997d). *Understanding the defiant child* (Videotape). New York: Guilford Press.

Barkley, R. A. (1998). *Attention-deficit/hyperactivity disorder: A handbook for diagnosis and treatment* (2nd ed.). New York: Guilford Press.

Barkley, R. A., Anastopoulos, A. D., Guevremont, D. G., & Fletcher, K. F. (1992). Adolescents with attention deficit hyperactivity disorder: Mother–adolescent interactions, family beliefs and conflicts, and maternal psychopathology. *Journal of Abnormal Child Psychology, 20*, 263–288.

Barkley, R. A., & Biederman, J. (1997). Towards a broader definition of the age of onset criterion for attention deficit hyperactivity disorder. *Journal of the American Academy of Child and Adolescent Psychiatry, 36*, 1204–1210.

Barkley, R. A., & Edelbrock, C. S. (1987). Assessing situational variation in children's behavior problems: The Home and School Situations Questionnaires. In R. Prinz (Ed.), *Advances in behavioral assessment of children and families* (Vol. 3, pp. 157–176). Greenwich, CT: JAI.

Barkley, R. A., Fischer, M., Edelbrock, C. S., & Smallish, L. (1990). The adolescent outcome of hyperactive children diagnosed by research criteria: I. An 8 year prospective follow-up study. *Journal of the American Academy of Child and Adolescent Psychiatry, 29,* 546–557.

Barkley, R. A., Fischer, M., Edelbrock, C. S., & Smallish, L. (1991). The adolescent outcome of hyperactive children diagnosed by research criteria: III. Mother–child interactions, family conflicts, and maternal psychopathology. *Journal of Child Psychology and Psychiatry, 32,* 233–256.

Barkley, R. A., Guevremont, D. G., Anastopoulos, A. D., & Fletcher, K. (1992). A comparison of three family therapy programs for treating family conflicts in adolescents with attention-deficit hyperactivity disorder. *Journal of Consulting and Clinical Psychology, 60,* 450–462.

Barkley, R. A., & Murphy, K. R. (1996). Psychological adjustment and adaptive impairments in young adults with ADHD. *Journal of Attention Disorders, 1,* 41–54.

Barkley, R. A., & Murphy, K. R. (1998). *Attention-deficit/hyperactivity disorder: A clinical handbook* (2nd ed.). New York: Guilford Press.

Bean, A. W., & Roberts, M. W. (1981). The effects of time-out release contingencies on changes in child noncompliance. *Journal of Abnormal Child Psychology, 9,* 95–105.

Beck, A. T., Steer, R. A., & Garbin, M. G. (1988). Psychometric properties of the Beck Depression Inventory: Twenty-five years of evaluation. *Clinical Psychology Review, 8,* 77–100.

Bell, R. Q., & Harper, L. V. (1977). *Child effects on adults.* Mahweh, NJ: Erlbaum.

Bernal, M. E., Klinnert, M. D., & Schultz, L. A. (1980). Outcome evaluation of behavioral parent training and client-centered parent counseling for children with conduct problems. *Journal of Applied Behavior Analysis, 13,* 677–691.

Biederman, J., Faraone, S. V., Keenan, K., & Tsuang, M. T. (1991). Evidence of a familial association between attention deficit disorder and major affective disorders. *Archives of General Psychiatry, 48,* 633–642.

Biederman, J., Faraone, S. V., Millberger, S., Curtis, S., Chen, L., Marrs, A., Ouellette, C., Moore, P., & Spencer, T. (1996). Predictors of persistence and remission of ADHD into adolescence: Results from a four-year prospective follow-up study. *Journal of the American Academy of Child and Adolescent, 35,* 343–351.

Biederman, J., Keenan, K., & Faraone, S. V. (1990). Parent-based diagnosis of attention deficit disorder predicts a diagnosis based on teacher report. *American Journal of Child and Adolescent Psychiatry, 29,* 698–701.

Blum, N. J., Williams, G. E., Friman, P. C., & Christophersen, E. R. (1995). Disciplining young children: The role of verbal instructions and reasoning. *Pediatrics, 96,* 336–341.

Braungart-Rieker, J., Rende, R. D., Plomin, R., DeFries, J. C., & Fulker, D. W. (1995). Genetic mediation of longitudinal associations between family environment and childhood behavior problems. *Development and Psychopathology, 7,* 233–245.

Breen, M. J., & Barkley, R. A. (1988). Child psychopathology and parenting stress in girls and boys having attention deficit disorder with hyperactivity. *Journal of Pediatric Psychology, 13,* 265–280.

Calvert, S. C., & McMahon, R. J. (1987). The treatment acceptability of a behavioral parent training program and its components. *Behavior Therapy, 2,* 165–179.

Capaldi, D. M. (1992). Co-occurrence of conduct problems and depressive symptoms in early adolescent boys: II. A 2-year follow-up at grade 8. *Development and Psychopathology, 4,* 125–144.

Conners, C. K. (1998). *The Conners Rating Scales.* North Tonawanda, NY: Multi-Health Systems.

Crits-Cristoph, P., & Mintz, J. (1991). Implications of therapist effects for the design and analysis of comparative studies of psychotherapies. *Journal of Consulting and Clinical Psychology, 59,* 20–26.

Dadds, M. R., & McHugh, T. A. (1992). Social support and treatment outcome in behavioral family therapy for child conduct problems. *Journal of Consulting and Clinical Psychology, 60,* 252–259.

Dadds, M. R., Schwartz, S., & Sanders, M. R. (1987). Marital discord and treatment outcome in behavioral treatment of child conduct disorders. *Journal of Consulting and Clinical Psychology, 55,* 396–403.

Danforth, J. S., Barkley, R. A., & Stokes, T. F. (1991). Observations of parent-child interactions with hyperactive children: Research and clinical implications. *Clinical Psychology Review, 11,* 703–727.

Dawkins, R. (1982). *The extended phenotype.* Oxford, England: Oxford University Press.

Day, D. E., & Roberts, M. W. (1982). An analysis of the physical punishment component of a parent training program. *Journal of Abnormal Child Psychology, 11,* 141–152.

Derogatis, L. (1986). *Manual for the Symptom Checklist 90—Revised (SCL-90-R).* Baltimore, MD: Author.

Dishion, T. J., & Andrews, D. W. (1995). Preventing escalation in problem behaviors with high-risk young adolescents: Immediate and 1-year outcomes. *Journal of Consulting and Clinical Psychology, 63,* 538–548.

Dishion, T. J., & Patterson, G. R. (1992). Age effects in parent training outcome. *Behavior Therapy, 23,* 719–729.

Dubey, D. R., O'Leary, S. G., & Kaufman, K. F. (1983). Training parents of hyperactive children in child management: A comparative outcome study. *Journal of Abnormal Child Psychology, 11,* 229–246.

Dumas, J. E. (1984). Interactional correlates of treatment outcome in behavioral parent training. *Journal of Consulting and Clinical Psychology, 52,* 946–954.

Dumas, J. E., & Wahler, R. G. (1983). Predictors of treatment outcome in parent training: Mother insularity and socioeconomic disadvantage. *Behavioral Assessment, 5,* 301–313.

Dumas, J. E., & Wahler, R. G. (1985). Indiscriminate mothering as a contextual factor in aggressive-oppositional child behavior: "Damned if you do and damned if you don't." *Journal of Abnormal Child Psychology, 13,* 1–17.

DuPaul, G. J., Anastopoulos, A. D., Power, T. J., Reid, R., Ikeda, M., & McGoey, K. (1998). Parent ratings of attention-deficit/hyperactivity disorder symptoms: Factor structure and normative data. *Journal of Psychopathology and Behavioral Assessment, 20,* 83–102.

DuPaul, G. J., & Barkley, R. A. (1992). Situational variability of attention problems: Psychometric properties of the Revised Home and School Situations Questionnaires. *Journal of Clinical Child Psychology, 21,* 178–188.

DuPaul, G. J., Barkley, R. A., & Connor, D. F. (1998). Stimulants. In R. A. Barkley, *Attention-deficit/hyperactivity disorder: A handbook for diagnosis and treatment* (2nd ed., pp. 510–551). New York: Guilford Press.

DuPaul, G. J., & Stoner, G. (1994). *ADHD in the schools: Assessment and intervention strategies.* New York: Guilford Press.

Elkins, I. J., McGue, M., & Iacono, W. G. (1997). Genetic and environmental influences on parent-son relationships: Evidence for increasing genetic influence during adolescence. *Developmental Psychology, 33,* 351–363.

Enyart, P. (1984). *Behavioral correlates of self-reported parent–adolescent relationship satisfaction.* Unpublished doctoral dissertation, West Virginia University, Morgantown.

Estrada, A. U., & Pinsof, W. M. (1995). The effectiveness of family therapies for selected behavioral disorders of childhood. *Journal of Marital and Family Therapy, 21,* 403–440.

Evans, S. W., Vallano, M.D., & Pelham, W. (1994). Treatment of parenting behavior with a psychostimulant: A case study of an adult with attention-deficit hyperactivity disorder. *Journal of Child and Adolescent Psychopharmacology, 4,* 63–69.

Eyberg, S. M., & Robinson, E. A. (1982). Parent-child interaction training: Effects on family functioning. *Journal of Clinical Child Psychology, 11,* 130–137.

Faraone, S. V., Biederman, J., Lehman, B., Keenan, K., Norman, D., Seidman, L. J., Kolodny, R., Krauss, I., Perrin, J., & Chen, W. (1993). Evidence for the independent familial transmission of attention deficit hyperactivity disorder and learning disabilities: Results from a family genetic study. *American Journal of Psychiatry, 150,* 891–895.

Farrington, D. P. (1995). The twelfth Jack Tizard memorial lecture: The development of offending and antisocial behavior from childhood—Key findings from the Cambridge study in delinquent development. *Journal of Child Psychology and Psychiatry, 360,* 929–964.

Fergusson, D. M., Horwood, L. J., & Lynskey, M. T, (1993). Prevalence and Comorbidity of DSM-III-R diagnoses in a birth cohort of 15 year olds. *Journal of the American Academy of Child and Adolescent Psychiatry, 32,* 1127–1133.

Firestone, P., Kelly, M. J., Goodman, J. T., & Davey, J. (1981). Differential effects of parent training and stimulant medication with hyperactives. *American Academy of Child Psychiatry, 20,* 135–147.

Firestone, P., & Witt, J. E. (1982). Characteristics of families completing and prematurely discontinuing a behavioral parent training program. *Journal of Pediatric Psychology, 7,* 209–222.

Fischer, M., Barkley, R. A., Fletcher, K., & Smallish, L. (1993). The stability of dimensions of behavior in ADHD and normal children over an 8 year period. *Journal of Abnormal Child Psychology, 21,* 315–337.

Fletcher, K., Fischer, M., Barkley, R. A., & Smallish, L. (1996). Sequential analysis of mother-adolescent interactions of ADHD, ADHD/ODD, and normal teenagers during neutral and conflict discussions. *Journal of Abnormal Child Psychology, 24,* 271–297.

Forehand, R. L., & McMahon, R. J. (1981). *Helping the noncompliant child: a clinician's guide to parent training.* New York: Guilford Press.

Forehand, R., & Scarboro, M. E. (1975). An analysis of children's oppositional behavior. *Journal of Abnormal Child Psychology, 3,* 27–31.

Foster, S. L., Prinz, R. J., & O'Leary, K. D. (1983). Impact on problem-solving communication training and generalization procedures on family conflict. *Child and Family Behavior Therapy, 5,* 1–23.

Frankel, F., & Simmons, J. Q., III. (1992). Parent behavioral training: Why and when some parents drop out. *Journal of Clinical Child Psychology, 21,* 322–330.

Frick, P. J., Lahey, B. B., Loeber, R, Stouthamer-Loeber, M., Christ, M. A., & Hanson, K. (1992). Familial risk factors to oppositional defiant disorder and conduct disorder: Parental psychopathology and maternal parenting. *Journal of Consulting and Clinical Psychology, 60,* 49–55.

Frick, P. J., Van Horn, Y., Lahey, B. B., Christ, M. A. G., Loeber, R., Hart, E. A., Tannenbaum, L., & Hanson, K. (1993). Oppositional defiant disorder and conduct disorder: A meta-analytic review of factor analyses and cross-validation in a clinic sample. *Clinical Psychology Review, 13,* 319–340.

Garfield, S. L., & Bergen, A. E. (Eds.). (1986). *Handbook of psychotherapy and behavior change* (3rd ed.). New York: Wiley.

Goldstein, A. P., Keller, H., & Erne, D. (1985). *Changing the abusive parent.* Champaign, IL: Research Press.

Goyette, C. H., Conners, C. K., & Ulrich, R. F. (1978). Normative data for Revised Conners Parent and Teacher Rating Scales. *Journal of Abnormal Child Psychology*, 6, 221–236.

Green, K. D., Forehand, R., & McMahon, R. J. (1979). Parental manipulation of compliance and noncompliance in normal and deviant children. *Behavior Modification*, 3, 245–266.

Greene, R. W., Biederman, J., Faraone, S. V., Ouellette, C. A., Penn, C., & Griffin, S. M. (1996). Toward a new psychometric definition of social disability in children with attention-deficit hyperactivity disorder. *Journal of American Academy of Child and Adolescent Psychiatry*, 35, 571–578.

Greenhill, L., & Osmon, B. B. (1991). *Ritalin*. New York: Mary Ann Liebert.

Haapasalo, J., & Tremblay, R. E. (1994). Physically aggressive boys from ages 6 to 12: Family background, parenting behavior, and prediction of delinquency. *Journal of Consulting and Clinical Psychology*, 62, 1044–1052.

Hersen, M., & Bellack, A. S. (Eds.). (1988). *Dictionary of behavioral assessment*. New York: Pergamon Press.

Hinshaw, S. P. (1987). On the distinction between attentional deficits/hyperactivity and conduct problems/aggression in child psychopathology. *Psychological Bulletin*, 101, 443–463.

Hinshaw, S. P. (1994). *Attention deficits and hyperactivity in children*. Thousand Oaks, CA: Sage.

Hinshaw, S. P., & Anderson, C. A. (1996). Conduct and oppositional defiant disorders. In E. J. Mash & R. A. Barkley (Eds.), *Child psychopathology* (pp. 113–152). New York: Guilford Press.

Hinshaw, S. P., Han, S. S., Erhardt, D., & Huber, A. (1992). Internalizing and externalizing behavior problems in preschool children: Correspondence among parent and teacher ratings and behavior observations. *Journal of Clinical Child Psychology*, 21, 143–150.

Holden, G. W., Lavigne, V. V., & Cameron, A. M. (1990). Probing the continuum of effectiveness in parent training: Characteristics of parents and preschoolers. *Journal of Clinical Child Psychology*, 19, 2–8.

Horn, W. F., Ialongo, N., Greenberg, G., Packard, T., & Smith-Winberry, C. (1990). Additive effects of behavioral parent training and self-control therapy with attention deficit hyperactivity disordered children. *Journal of Clinical Child Psychology*, 19, 98–110.

Horn, W. F., Ialongo, N. S., Pascoe, J. M., Greenberg, G., Packard, T., Lopez, M., Wagner, A., & Puttler, L. (1991). Additive effects of psychostimulants, parent training, and self-control therapy with ADHD children. *Journal of American Academy of Child and Adolescent Psychiatry*, 30, 233–240.

Horn, W. F., Ialongo, N., Popovich, S., & Peradotto, D. (1987). Behavioral parent training and cognitive-behavioral self-control therapy with ADD-H children: comparative and combined effects. *Journal of Clinical Child Psychology*, 16, 57–68.

Humphreys, L., Forehand, R., McMahon, R., & Roberts, M. (1978). Parent behavioral training to modify child noncompliance: Effects on untreated siblings. *Journal of Behavioral Therapy and Experimental Psychiatry*, 9, 1–5.

Jensen, P. S., Watanabe, H. K., Richters, J. E., Cortes, R., Roper, M., & Liu, S. (1995). Prevalence of mental disorder in military children and adolescents: Findings from a two-stage community survey. *Journal of American Academy of Child and Adolescent Psychiatry*, 34, 1514–1524.

Johnson, S. M., Wahl, G., Martin, S., & Johansson, S. (1973). How deviant is the normal child? A behavioral analysis of the preschool child and his family. In R. D. Rubin, J. P. Brady, & J. D. Henderson (Eds.), *Advances in behavior therapy* (Vol. 4). New York: Academic Press.

Johnston, C. (1992, February). *The influence of behavioral parent training on inattentive overactive and aggressive-defiant behaviors in ADHD children*. Paper presented at the annual meeting of the Society for Research in Child and Adolescent Psychopathology, Irvine, CA.

Johnston, C. (1996). Parent characteristics and parent-child interactions in families of nonproblem children and ADHD children with higher and lower levels of oppositional-defiant behavior. *Journal of Abnormal Child Psychology, 24,* 85–104.

Kazdin, A. E. (1980). Acceptability of time out from reinforcement procedures for disruptive child behavior. *Behavior Therapy, 11,* 329–344.

Kazdin, A. E. (1991). Effectiveness of psychotherapy with children and adolescents. *Journal of Consulting and Clinical Psychology, 58,* 729–740.

Kazdin, A. E., Esveldt-Dawson, K., French, N. H., & Unis, A. S. (1987). Effects of parent management training and problem-solving skills training combined in the treatment of antisocial child behavior. *American Academy of Child and Adolescent Psychiatry, 26,* 416–424.

Keenan, K., & Shaw D. S. (1994). The development of aggression in toddlers: A study of low-income families. *Journal of Abnormal Child Psychology, 22,* 53–77.

Kelley, M. L. (1990). *School–home notes: Promoting children's classroom success.* New York: Guilford Press.

Kelley, M. L., Embry, L. H., & Baer, D. M. (1979). Skills for child management and family support. *Behavior Modification, 3,* 373–396.

Knapp, P. A., & Deluty, R. H. (1989) Relative effectiveness of two behavioral parent training programs. *Journal of Clinical Child Psychology, 18,* 314–322.

Lachar, D. (1982). *Personality Inventory for Children (PIC): Revised Format Manual Supplement.* Los Angeles: Western Psychological Services.

Lahey, B. B., Appelgate, B., Barkley, R. A., Garfinkel, B., McBurnett, K., Lerdyk, L., Greenhill, L., Hynd, G. W., Frick, P. J., Newcorn, J., Biederman, J., Ollendick, T., Hart, E. L., Perez, D., Waldman, I., & Shaffer, D. (1994). DSM-IV field trials for oppositional defiant disorder and conduct disorder in children and adolescents. *American Journal of Psychiatry, 151,* 1163–1171.

Lahey, B. B., Appelgate, B., McBurnett, K. Biederman, J., Greenhill, L., Hynd, G. W., Barkley, R. A., Mewcorn, J., Jensem, P., Richters, J., Garfinkel, B., Kerdyk, L., Frick, P. J., Ollendick, T., Perez, D., Hart, E., Waldman, I., & Shaffer, D. (1994). DSM-IV field trials for attention deficit hyperactivity disorder in children and adolescents. *American Journal of Psychiatry, 151,* 1673–1685.

Lahey, B. B., & Loeber, R. (1994). Framework for a developmental model of oppositional defiant disorder and conduct disorder. In D. K. Routh (Ed.), *Disruptive behavior disorders in childhood* (pp. 139–180). New York: Plenum Press.

Lahey, B. B., Loeber, R., Quay, H. C., Frick, P. J., & Grimm, J. (1992). Oppositional defiant and conduct disorders: Issues to be resolved for DSM-IV. *Journal of American Academy of Child and Adolescent Psychiatry, 31,* 539–546.

Lahey, B. B., Piacentini, J. C., McBurnett, K., Stone, P., Hartdagen, S., & Hynd, G. W. (1988). Psychopathology in the parents of children with conduct disorder and hyperactivity. *Journal of the American Academy of Child and Adolescent Psychiatry, 27,* 163–170.

Latham, P., & Latham, R. (1992). *ADD and the law.* Washington, DC: JKL Communications.

Lewinsohn, P. M., Hops, H., Roberts, R. E., Seeley, J. R., & Andrews, J. A. (1993). Adolescent psychopathology: I. Prevalence and incidence of depression and other DSM-III-R disorders in high school students. *Journal of Abnormal Psychology, 102,* 133–144.

Lilienfeld, S. O., & Marino, L. (1995). Mental disorder as a Roschian concept: A critique of Wakefield's "harmful dysfunction" analysis. *Journal of Abnormal Psychology, 104,* 411–420.

Little, L. M., & Kelley, M. L. (1989). The efficacy of response cost procedures for reducing children's noncompliance to parental instructions. *Behavior Therapy, 20,* 515–534.

Locke, H. J., & Wallace, K. M. (1959). Short marital adjustment and prediction tests: Their reliability and validity. *Journal of Marriage and Family Living, 21,* 251–255.

Loeber, R. (1988). Natural histories of conduct problems, delinquency, and associated substance use. In B. B. Lahey & A. E. Kazdin (Eds.), *Advances in clinical child psychology* (Vol. 11). New York: Plenum Press.

Loeber, R. (1990). Development and risk factors of juvenile antisocial behavior and delinquency. *Clinical Psychology Review, 10,* 1–41.

Loeber, R., Green, S. M., Lahey, B. B., Christ, M. A. G., & Frick, P. J. (1992). Developmental sequences in the age of onset of disruptive child behaviors. *Journal of Child and Family Studies, 1,* 21–41.

Loeber, R., Green, S., Lahey, B. B., & Stouthamer-Loeber, M. (1991). Differences and similarities between children, mothers, and teachers as informants on disruptive behavior disorders. *Journal of Abnormal Child Psychology, 19,* 75–95.

Loeber, R., Wung, P., Keenan, K., Giroux, B., Stouthamer-Loeber, M., Van Kammen, W. B, & Maughan, B. (1993). Developmental pathways in disruptive child behavior. *Developmental and Psychopathology, 5,* 101–131.

Lynskey, M. T., & Fergusson, D. M. (1994). Childhood conduct problems, attention deficit behaviors, and adolescent alcohol, tobacco, and illicit drug use. *Journal of Abnormal Child Psychology, 23,* 281–302.

Mann, B. J., Borduin, C. M., Henggeler, S. W., & Blaske, D. M. (1990). An investigation of systemic conceptualizations of parent-child coalitions and symptom change. *Journal of Consulting and Clinical Psychology, 3,* 336–344.

Mann, B. J., & MacKenzie, E. P. (1996). Pathways among marital functioning, parental behaviors, and child behavior problems in school-age boys. *Journal of Clinical Child Psychology, 25,* 183–191.

Markel, G., & Greenbaum, J. (1996). *Performance breakthroughs for adolescents with learning disabilities or ADD.* Champaign, IL: Research Press.

Mash, E. J., & Barkley, R. A. (Eds.). (1996). *Child psychopathology.* New York: Guilford Press.

Mash, E. J., & Barkley, R. A. (Eds.). (1998). *Treatment of childhood disorders* (2nd ed.). New York: Guilford Press.

Mash, E. J., & Dozois, D. J. A. (1996). Child psychopathology: A developmental systems perspective. In E. J. Mash & R. A. Barkley (Eds.), *Child psychopathology* (pp. 3–62). New York: Guilford Press.

Mash, E. J., & Johnston, C. (1982). A comparison of mother–child interactions of younger and older hyperactive and normal children. *Child Development, 53,* 1371–1381.

Mash, E. J., & Terdal, L. G. (Eds.). (1997). *Assessment of childhood disorders* (3rd ed.). New York: Guilford Press.

McGee, R., Feehan, M., Williams, S., Partridge, F., Silva, P. A., & Kelly, J. (1990). DSM-III disorders in a large sample of adolescents. *American Academy of Child and Adolescent Psychiatry, 29,* 611–619.

McMahon, R. J., & Forehand, R. (1984). Parent training for the noncompliant child. In R. F. Dangel & R. A. Polster (Eds.), *Parent training: Foundations of research and practice.* New York: Guilford Press.

McMahon, R. J., & Wells, K. C. (1998). Conduct problems. In E. J. Mash & R. A. Barkley (Eds.), *Treatment of childhood disorders* (2nd ed., pp. 111–209). New York: Guilford Press.

Moffitt, T. E. (1990). Juvenile delinquency and attention deficit disorder: Boys' developmental trajectories from age 3 to age 15. *Child Development, 61,* 893–910.

Murphy, K. R., & Barkley, R. A. (1996a). Parents of children with attention-deficit/hyperactivity disorder: Psychological and attentional impairment. *American Journal of Orthopsychiatry*, *66*, 93–102.

Murphy, K. R., & Barkley, R. A. (1996b). Prevalence of DSM-IV ADHD symptoms in an adult community sample of licensed drivers. *Journal of Attention Disorders*, *1*, 147–161.

Olson, S. L. (1992). Development of conduct problems and peer rejection in preschool children: A social systems analysis. *Journal of Abnormal Child Psychology*, *20*, 327–350.

Olweus, D. (1979). Stability of aggressive reaction patterns in males: A review. *Psychological Bulletin*, *86*, 852–875.

Olweus, D. (1980). Familial and temperamental determinants of aggressive behavior in adolescent boys: A causal analysis. *Developmental Psychology*, *16*, 644–660.

Paternite, C., & Loney, J. (1980). Childhood hyperkinesis: Relationships between symptomatology and home environment. In C. K. Whalen & B. Henker (Eds.), *Hyperactive children: The social ecology of identification and treatment*. New York: Academic Press.

Patterson, G. R. (1976). The aggressive child: victim and architect of a coercive system. In E. J. Mash, L. A. Hamerlynck, & L. C. Handy (Eds.), *Behavior modification and families* (pp. 267–316). New York: Brunner/Mazel.

Patterson, G. R. (1982). *Coercive family process*. Eugene, OR: Castalia.

Patterson, G. R., & Chamberlain, P. (1992). A functional analysis of resistance. *Clinical Psychology: Science and Practice*, *1*, 53–70.

Patterson, G. R., Chamberlain, P., & Reid, J. B. (1982). A comparative evaluation of a parent-training program. *Behavior Therapy*, *13*, 638–650.

Patterson, G. R., Dishion, T. J., & Chamberlain, P. (1993). Outcomes and methodological issues relating to treatment of antisocial children. In T. R. Giles (Ed.), *Handbook of effective psychotherapy*. New York: Plenum Press.

Patterson, G. R., & Fleischman, M. J. (1979). Maintenance of treatment effects: some considerations concerning family systems and follow-up data. *Behavior Therapy*, *10*, 168–185.

Patterson, G. R., & Forgatch, M. S. (1985). Therapist behavior as a determinant for client noncompliance: A paradox for the behavior modifier. *Journal of Consulting and Clinical Psychology*, *53*, 846–851.

Patterson, G. R., Reid, J. B., & Dishion, T. J. (1992). *Antisocial boys*. Eugene, OR: Castalia.

Pearson, J. L., Ialongo, N. S., Hunter, A. G., & Kellam, S. G. (1993). Family structure and aggressive behavior in a population of urban elementary school children. *Journal of American Academy of Child and Adolescent Psychiatry*, *33*, 540–548.

Pelham, W. E., Jr., Gnagy, E. M., Greenslade, K. E., & Milich, R. (1992). Teacher ratings of DSM-III symptoms for the disruptive behavior disorders. *Journal of the American Academy of Child and Adolescent Psychiatry*, *31*, 210–218.

Pelham, W. E., & Lang, A. R. (1993). Parental alcohol consumption and deviant child behavior: Laboratory studies of reciprocal effects. *Clinical Psychology Review*, *13*, 763–784.

Pfiffner, L. J., Jouriles, E. N., Brown, M. M., Etscheidt, M. A., & Kelly, J. A. (1988). *Enhancing the effects of parent training for single-parent families*. Paper presented at the 22nd annual Association for Advancement of Behavior Therapy Convention, New York.

Pike, A., McGuire, S., Hetherington, M. E., Reiss, D., & Plomin, R. (1996). Family environment and adolescent depressive symptoms and antisocial behavior: A multivariate genetic analysis. *Developmental Psychology*, *32*, 590–603.

Pike, A., Reiss, D., Hetherington, E. M., & Plomin, R. (1996). Using MZ differences in the search for nonshared environmental effects. *Journal of Child Psychology and Psychiatry*, *37*, 695–704.

Pisterman, S., McGrath, P., Firestone, P., Goodman, J. T., Webster, I., & Mallory, R. (1989). Outcome of parent-mediated treatment of preschoolers with attention deficit disorder with hyperactivity. *Journal of Consulting and Clinical Psychology, 57*, 628–635.

Plomin, R. (1995). Genetics and children's experiences in the family. *Journal of Child Psychology and Psychiatry, 36*, 33–68.

Pollard, S., Ward, E., & Barkley, R. (1983). The effects of parent training and Ritalin on the parent–child interactions of hyperactive boys. *Child and Family Behavior Therapy, 5*, 51–69.

Prior, M. (1992). Childhood temperament. *Journal of Child Psychology and Psychiatry, 33*, 249–279.

Prinz, R. J., & Miller, G. E. (1994). Family-based treatment for childhood antisocial behavior: Experimental influences on dropout and engagement. *Journal of Consulting and Clinical Psychology, 62*, 645–650.

Quici, F. L., Wheeler, S. R., & Bolle, J. (1996, March). *Does training parents of defiant children really work?: Seven years of data.* Paper presented at The National Association of School Psychologists Annual Convention, Atlanta, GA.

Rapport, M. D., & Kelly, K. L. (1993). Psychostimulant effects on learning and cognitive function in children with attention deficit hyperactivity disorder: Findings and implications. In J. L. Matson (Ed.), *Hyperactivity in children: A handbook* (pp. 97–136). New York: Pergamon.

Reynolds, C., & Kamphaus, R. (1994). *Behavioral Assessment System for Children.* Circle Pines, MN: American Guidance Systems.

Richters, J. E., & Cichetti, D. (1993). Mark Twain meets DSM-III-R: Conduct disorder, development, and the concept of harmful dysfunction. *Development and Psychopathology, 5*, 5–29.

Roberts, M. W. (1985). Praising child compliance: Reinforcement or ritual? *Journal of Abnormal Child Psychology, 13*, 611–629.

Roberts, M. W., Hatzenbuehler, L. C., & Bean, A. W. (1981). The effects of differential attention and time out on child noncompliance. *Behavior Therapy, 12*, 93–99.

Roberts, M. W., McMahon, R. J., Forehand, R., & Humphreys, L. (1978). The effect of parental instruction-giving on child compliance. *Behavior Therapy, 9*, 793–798.

Robin, A. L. (1981). A controlled evaluation of problem-solving communication training with parent–adolescent conflict. *Behavior Therapy, 12*, 593–609.

Robin, A. L. (1998). *ADHD in adolescents: Diagnosis and treatment.* New York: Guilford Press.

Robin, A. L., & Foster, S. L. (1984). Problem solving communication training: A behavioral–family systems approach to parent–adolescent conflict. In P. Karoly & J. J. Steffen (Eds.), *Adolescent behavior disorders: Foundations and contemporary concerns* (pp. 195–240). Lexington, MA: Heath.

Robin, A. L., & Foster, S. (1989). *Negotiating parent–adolescent conflict: A behavioral–family systems approach.* New York: Guilford Press.

Robin, A. L., Koepke, T., & Moye, A. (1990). Multidimensional assessment of parent-adolescent relations. *Psychological Assessment: A Journal of Consulting and Clinical Psychology, 2*, 451–459.

Rogers, T. R., Forehand, R., Griest, D. L, Wells, K. C., & McMahon, R. J. (1981). Socioeconomic status: effects of parent and child behaviors and treatment outcome of parent training. *Journal of Clinical Child Psychology, 10*, 98–101.

Roizen, N. J., Blondis, T. A., Irwin, M., & Stein, M. (1994). Adaptive functioning in children with attention-deficit hyperactivity disorder. *Archives of Pediatric and Adolescent Medicine, 148*, 1137–1142.

Rowe, D. (1994). *The limits of family influence.* New York: Guilford Press.

Russo, D. C., Cataldo, M. F., & Cushing, P. J. (1981). Compliance training and behavioral covariation in the treatment of multiple behavior problems. *Journal of Applied Behavior Analysis, 14,* 209–222.

Salzinger, S., Kaplan, S., & Artemyeff, C. (1983). Mothers' personal social networks and child maltreatment. *Journal of Abnormal Psychology, 92,* 68–76.

Sanders, M. R. (1996). New directions in behavioral family intervention with children. In T. H. Ollendick & R. J. Prinz (Eds.), *Advances in clinical child psychology* (Vol. 18, pp. 283–330). New York: Plenum Press.

Sanders, M. R., & Christensen, A. P. (1984). A comparison of the effects of child management and planned activities training in five parenting environments. *Journal of Abnormal Child Psychology, 13,* 101–117.

Sanders, M. R., & Dadds, M. R. (1982). The effects of planned activities and child management procedures in parent training: An analysis of setting generally. *Behavior Therapy, 13,* 452–461.

Sanders, M. R., & Glynn, T. (1981). Training parents in behavioral self-management: An analysis of generalization and maintenance. *Journal of Applied Behavior Analysis, 14,* 223–237.

Scarr, S. (1992). Developmental theories for the 1990s: Development and individual differences. *Child Development, 63,* 1–19.

Scarr, S., & McCartney, K. (1983). How people make their own environments: A theory of genotype–environment effects. *Child Development, 54,* 424–435.

Schachar, R., & Wachsmuth, R. (1990). Oppositional disorder in children: A validation study comparing conduct disorder, oppositional disorder and normal control children. *Journal of Child Psychology and Psychiatry, 31,* 1089–1102.

Schubiner, H. (1995). *ADHD in adolescence: Our point of view* (Videotape). Detroit, MI: Children's Hospital of Michigan Department of Educational Services.

Shaw, D. S., & Vondra, J. I. (1995). Infant attachment security and maternal predictors of early behavior problems: A longitudinal study of low-income families. *Journal of Abnormal Child Psychology, 23,* 335–357.

Shekim, W., Asarnow, R. F., Hess, E., Zaucha, K., & Wheeler, N. (1990). An evaluation of attention deficit disorder—residual type. *Comprehensive Psychiatry, 31,* 416–425.

Shriver, M. D., & Allen, K. D. (1996). The time-out grid: A guide to effective discipline. *School Psychology Quarterly, 11,* 67–75.

Sleator, E. K., & Ullmann, R. K. (1981). Can the physician diagnose hyperactivity in the office? *Pediatrics, 67,* 13–17.

Snyder, J., & Brown, K. (1983). Oppositional behavior and noncompliance in preschool children: Environmental correlates and skills deficits. *Behavioral Assessment, 5,* 333–348.

Snyder, J., & Patterson, G. R. (1995). Individual differences in social aggression: A test of reinforcement model of socialization in the natural environment. *Behavior Therapy, 26,* 371–391.

Spaccarelli, S., Cotler, S., & Penman, D. (1992). Problem-solving skills training as a supplement to behavioral parent training. *Cognitive Therapy and Research, 16,* 1–18.

Speltz, M. L., DeKlyen, M., Greenberg, M. T., & Dryden, M. (1995). Clinic referral for oppositional defiant disorder: Relative significance of attachment and behavioral variables. *Journal of Abnormal Child Psychology, 23,* 487–507.

Spitzer, A., Webster-Stratton, C. & Hollinsworth, T. (1991). Coping with conduct-problem children: Parents gaining knowledge and control. *Journal of Clinical Child Psychology, 20,* 413–427.

Stormont-Spurgin, M., & Zentall, S. S. (1995). Contributing factors in the manifestation of aggression in preschoolers with hyperactivity. *Journal of Child Psychology and Psychiatry, 3*, 491–509.

Strain, P. S., Steele, P., Ellis, T., & Timm, M. A. (1982). Long-term effects of oppositional child treatment with mothers as therapists and therapist trainers. *Journal of Applied Behavior Analysis, 15*, 163–169.

Strain, P. S., Young, C. C., & Horowitz, J. (1981). Generalized behavior change during oppositional child training: An examination of child and family demographic variables. *Behavior Modification, 5*, 15–26.

Strayhorn, J. M., & Weidman, C. S. (1989). Reduction of attention deficit and internalizing symptoms in preschoolers through parent-child interaction training. *American Academy of Child and Adolescent Psychiatry, 28*, 888–896.

Strayhorn, J. M., & Weidman, C. S. (1991). Follow-up one year after parent–child interaction training: effects on behavior of preschool children. *Journal of the American Academy of Child and Adolescent Psychiatry, 30*, 138–143.

Swanson, J. M., McBurnett, K., Christian, D. L., & Wigal, T. (1995). Stimulant medications and the treatment of children with ADHD. In T. H. Ollendick & R. J. Prinz (Ed.), *Advances in clinical child psychology* (Vol. 17, pp. 265–321). New York: Plenum Press.

Tolan, P. H. (1987). Implications of age of onset for delinquency risk. *Journal of Abnormal Child Psychology, 15*, 47–65.

Tremblay, R. E., Masse, B., Perron, D., Leblanc, M., Schwartzman, A. E., & Ledingham, J. E. (1992). Early disruptive behavior, poor school achievement, delinquent behavior, and delinquent personality: Longitudinal analyses. *Journal of Consulting and Clinical Psychology, 60*, 65–72.

Tremblay, R. E., Pihl, R. O., Vitaro, F., & Dobkin, P. L. (1994). Predicting early onset of male antisocial behavior from preschool behavior. *Archives of General Psychiatry, 51*, 732–738.

Tschann, J. M., Kaiser, P. Chesney, M. A., Alkon, A., & Boyce, W. T. (1996). Resilience and vulnerability among preschool children: Family functioning, temperament, and behavior problems. *Journal of the American Academy of Child and Adolescent Psychiatry, 35*, 184–191.

Vaden-Kiernan, N., Ialongo, N. S., Pearson, J., & Kellam, S. (1995). Household family structure and children's aggressive behavior, a longitudinal study of urban elementary school children. *Journal of Abnormal Child Psychology, 23*, 553–568.

Vasta, R. (1981). On token rewards and real dangers: A look at the data. *Behavior Modification, 5*, 129–140.

Vuchinich, S., Bank, L., & Patterson, G. R. (1992). Parenting, peers, and the stability of antisocial behavior in preadolescent boys. *Developmental Psychology, 28*, 510–521.

Wahler, R. (1975). Some structural aspects of deviant child behavior. *Journal of Applied Behavior Analysis, 8*, 27–42.

Wahler, R. G. (1980). The insular mother: Her problems in parent–child treatment. *Journal of Applied Behavior Analysis, 13*, 207–219.

Wahler, R. G., & Afton, A. D. (1980.) Attentional processes in insular and noninsular mothers: Some differences in their summary reports about child problem behaviors. *Child Behavior Therapy, 2*, 25–41.

Wahler, R. G., Cartor, P. G., Fleischman, J., & Lambert, W. (1993). The impact of synthesis teaching and parent training with mothers of conduct-disordered children. *Journal of Abnormal Child Psychology, 21*, 425–440.

Wahler, R. G., & Fox, J. J. (1980). Solitary toy play and time out: A family treatment package for children with aggressive and oppositional behavior. *Journal of Applied Behavior Analysis, 13*, 23–39.

Wahler, R. G., & Graves. M. G. (1983). Setting events in social networks: Ally or enemy in child behavior therapy? *Behavior Therapy, 14*, 19–36.

Wakefield, J. C. (1992). Disorder as harmful dysfunction: A conceptual critique of DSM-III-R's definition of mental disorder. *Psychological Review, 99*, 232–247.

Webster-Stratton, C. (1982). The long-term effects of a videotape modeling parent-training program: Comparison of immediate and 1-year follow up results. *Behavior Therapy, 13*, 702–714.

Webster-Stratton, C., & Hammond, M. (1990). Predictors of treatment outcome in parent training for families with conduct problem children. *Behavior Therapy, 21*, 319–337.

Webster-Stratton, C., Hollinsworth, T., & Kolpacoff, M. (1989). The long-term effectiveness and clinical significance of three cost-effective training programs for families with conduct-problem children. *Journal of Consulting and Clinical Psychology, 57*, 550–553.

Webster-Stratton, C., Kolpacoff, M., & Hollinsworth, T. (1995). Self-administered videotape therapy for families with conduct-problem children: Comparison with two cost-effective treatments and a control group. *Journal of Consulting and Clinical Psychology, 56*, 558–566.

Webster-Stratton, C., & Spitzer, A. (1996). Parenting a young child with conduct problems. In T. H. Ollendick & R. J. Prinz (Ed.), *Advances in clinical child psychology* (Vol. 18, pp. 1–62). New York: Plenum Press.

Weiss, G. (1992). *Child and adolescent psychiatry clinics of North America: Attention-deficit hyperactivity disorder*. Philadelphia: W. B. Saunders.

Weiss, G., & Hechtman, L. T. (1993). *Hyperactive children grown up* (2nd ed.): *ADHD in children, adolescents, and adults*. New York: Guilford Press.

Wells, K. C., & Forehand, R. (1985). Conduct and oppositional disorders. In P. H. Bornstein & A. E. Kazdin (Eds.), *Handbook of clinical behavior therapy with children* (pp. 219–265). Champaign, IL: Dorsey Press.

Wells, K. C., Forehand, R., & Griest, D. L. (1980). Generality of treatment effects from treated to untreated behaviors resulting from a parent training program. *Journal of Clinical Child Psychology, 9*, 217–219.

Wenning, K., Nathan, P., & King, S. (1993). Mood disorders in children with oppositional defiant disorder: A pilot study. *American Journal of Orthopsychiatry, 63*, 295–299.

Werry, J., & Aman, M. (1998). *Practitioners guide to psychoactive drugs with children and adolescents*. New York: Plenum Press.

Williams, C. A., & Forehand, R. (1984). An examination of predictor variables for child compliance and noncompliance. *Journal of Abnormal Child Psychology, 12*, 491–504.

Wozniak, J., & Biederman, J. (1995). Prepubertal mania exists (and co-exists with ADHD). *ADHD Report, 2*(3), 5–6.

Zoccolillo, M. (1993). Gender and the development of conduct disorder. *Development and Psychopathology, 5*, 65–78.

# Index

ADHD; *see* Attention-Deficit/
    Hyperactivity Disorder
Adolescent(s)
    assessment of; *see* Assessment
    interviewing, 53–54
    involving in problem
        solving, 77
    one-on-one time with, 97–98
    PSCT indicated for, 2–3
    psychological characteristics
        of, 88–89
    psychological strengths and
        weaknesses of, 45–46
Adult Behavior Rating Scale
    Self-Report of Childhood
        Behavior, 195
    Self-Report of Current
        Behavior, 194
Advocacy, school, 119–124
    parent handout for, 212
Aggressive behavior, parental,
    34–35
Anxiety/mood disorders
    adolescent, 53–54
    evaluation questions, 178–
        189
Argument, anatomy of, 25–27,
    28*f*
Asperger's Disorder, 49
Assessment, 44–71
    adolescent interview in, 53–
        54
    for comorbid conditions, 45

culture-sensitive, 45
differential diagnosis in, 44–
    45
legal and ethical issues, 67–69
materials for, 157–198
    Adult Behavior Rating
        Scale, 194–195
    child and family informa-
        tion form, 162
    developmental and
        medical history form,
        163–165
    Disruptive Behavior
        Disorders Rating Scale
        (Parents), 166–167
    Disruptive Behavior
        Disorders Rating Scale
        (Teachers), 168–193
    Issues Checklist for
        Parents and Teenagers,
        196–198
    questionnaire instructions,
        160–161
methods for, 46–66
    adolescent behavior rating
        scales, 55–57
    adolescent interview, 53–
        54
    family conflict ratings,
        58–62
    parental interview, 47–53
    peer relationship methods,
        58

preceding evaluation, 46–
    47
self-report rating scales
    (children), 57–58
self-report rating scales
    (parents), 62–66
teacher interview, 54–55
parental interview in, 47–53
of parental training potential,
    69–70
for psychological strengths
    and weaknesses, 45–46
purposes of, 44–46
teacher interview in, 54–55
treatment implications of,
    66–67
Attending skills, parental, 100–
    103
Attention, positive
developing, 95–99
    parent handout for develop-
        ing, 205–206
Attention-Deficit/Hyperactivity
    Disorder, 1
criteria for, 23*t*, 50–51
discussing with parents, 83–
    86
DSM-IV summation scores
    for, 64, 65*t*, 66*t*
educational rights of children
    with, 123
federal memorandum on,
    213–218

evaluation questions, 176–
178
family reaction to diagnosis
of, 85–86
government protections and
entitlements and, 68
laboratory measures of, 44
medications for, 7
with ODD and/or CD, 20
parental, 63–64, 89
temperament/cognitive
factors in, 37
treatment justification
criteria, 39–43
Atypical Pervasive Developmental Disorders, 6, 49

**B**

Back-handed compliments, 33
BASC; *see* Behavioral Assessment System for Children
Behavior(s)
anticipating, 90–91
developmentally inappropri-
ate/statistically deviant,
40
disruptive, meta-analysis of
studies on, 19*f*
emotional distress due to, 41
impairment-producing, 41
negative, 32; *see also* specific
behavior disorders
positive, parental failure to
reinforce, 32–34
Behavior cycle, coercive, 93–
94
parent handout for, 204
Behavior management; *see also*
Family-management
practices
ABC's of, 90
parent handout for, 203
principles of, 72–75, 87–
94
Behavior rating scales
adolescent, 55–57
children's self-report, 57–58
for family conflict, 58–62
parents' self-report, 62–66
for peer relationships, 58

Behavioral Assessment System
for Children, 46
source for, 55
Behavioral contracts
completion of, 113–115
establishing, 104–108
point system for, 106–107
sample form, 208
Beliefs, unreasonable
adolescent handout for, 230–
231
dealing with, 145–152
parent handout for, 226–229
Bipolar Disorder, 49
evaluation questions for,
187–188

**C**

CBCL; *see* Child Behavior
Checklist
CD; *see* Conduct Disorder
Child(ren)
psychological and social
strengths of, evaluation
questions, 191
report liability of, 53–54
Child Attention Problems
Scale, 57
Child Behavior Checklist, 46
source for, 55
Childhood disorders, DSM,
review of, 173–178
Children's Atypical Development Scale, 49
Coercive behavior cycle, 93–94
parent handout for, 204
Cognitive factors
parental, 38
teen defiance and, 37
Commands, effective, 102–103
parent handout for, 207
Communication skills; *see also*
Problem-solving commu-
nication training
introduction to, 139–142
parent handout for, 225
practicing, 143–144
Compliance, praising, 102
Compliments, back-handed,
33

Conduct Disorder, 2; *see also*
Oppositional Defiant and
Conduct Disorder
criteria for, 22*t,* 50–51
evaluation questions, 174–176
ODD association with, 20
pathways leading to, 20–21
Conners Parent and Teacher
Rating Scales, 56
Consequences
consistency of, 73–74, 92
immediacy of, 72, 92
inconsistency of, 32–33, 33–
34
positive versus negative, 91
predictability of, 73
specificity of, 73, 91–92
well-balanced, 92–93
Contingency-management
system, 105–107
Contracts, behavioral; *see*
Behavioral contracts

**D**

DBDRS; *see* Disruptive Behavior Disorders Rating Scale
Defiance/noncompliance; *see also*
Oppositional Defiant and
Conduct Disorder
adolescent temperament and
cognitive factors in, 37
assessment of; *see* Assessment
causes of, 36–39
clinic referrals for, 24–25
contextual factors in, 38–39
defined, 18
developmental persistence of,
30
differential diagnosis of, 44–45
family conflict and, 25–27,
26*f*
family social ecology and,
28–30, 29*f*
impaired child–family-
management practices
and, 37
negative developmental outcomes and, 30*t,* 30–31
parental temperament and
cognitive factors in, 38

Defiance/noncompliance
    (*continued*)
    pervasiveness of, 28
    prevalence of, 21–22, 24
    rationale for focus on, 24–31
    research on, 31–36
    and treatment of other
        problems, 31
Depression
    adolescent, 53–54
    parental, 65–66
Depressive Disorder, evaluation
    questions for, 186
*Diagnostic and Statistical Manual
    of Mental Disorders* (4th ed.)
    ADHD criteria of, 50–51
    ADHD summation scores,
        64, 65*t*, 66*t*
    CD criteria of, 50–51
    field trial limitations of, 50–
        51
    ODD criteria of, 20, 50–51
    review of childhood disor-
        ders, 173–178
Disruptive Behavior Disorder,
    evaluation questions for,
    176
Disruptive Behavior Disorders
    Rating Scale, 46, 56
    Parent Form, 166–167
    Teacher Form, 168–193
Dysthymic Disorder, evaluation
    questions for, 184–185


E

Environmental factors, conflict
    and, 38–39
Ethical issues, 67–69
Ethnic background, norms for, 45
Expectations, unreasonable,
    dealing with,
    145–149


F

Family(ies)
    demographic data on, 48
    evaluation form, 162
    PSCT indicated for, 2–3

reciprocal interactions in, 75
respecting structure of, 78–
    79
social ecology of, teen
    defiance and, 28–30,
    29*f*
stress of, 89–90
Family conflict
    ratings of, 58–62
    teen defiance and, 25–27,
        26*f*
Family history, evaluation
    questions for, 191–193
Family-management practices;
    *see also* Behavior manage-
    ment
    deficient, 36–37
    evaluation questions, 189
Family training program
    behavior-management
        principles in, 72–
        75
    handouts for, 199–231
        Step 2, 203–204
        Step 3, 205–206
        Step 4, 207
        Step 5, 208–210
        Step 8, 211
        Step 9, 212–218
        Step 10, 219–224
        Step 13, 225
        Step 15, 226–231
    justification for, 39–43
    overview of, 72–78
    sequence of steps, 79
    Step 1: discussion of ADHD
        and ODD, 83–86
    Step 2: behavior-manage-
        ment principles, 87–
        94
    Step 3: developing positive
        attention, 95–99
    Step 4: developing parental
        attending skills, 100–
        103
    Step 5: establishing behav-
        ioral contract, 104–
        108
    Step 6: usung response cost,
        109–112

Step 7: completing the
    contracts/point system,
    113–115
Step 8: grounding, 116–118
Step 9: school advocacy,
    119–124
Step 10: PSCT, 125–132
Step 11: practicing problem
    solving, 133–135
Step 12: practicing problem
    solving (cont'd), 136–
    138
Step 13: intro to communica-
    tion skills, 139–142
Step 14: practicing communi-
    cation skills, 143–144
Step 15: dealing with
    unreasonable beliefs/
    expectations, 145–
    149
Step 16: catching unreason-
    able beliefs, 150–152
Step 17: more family
    practice, 153–154
Step 18: concluding treat-
    ment, 155–156


G

Generalized Anxiety Disorder,
    evaluation questions for,
    182–183
Genetic factors, family conflict
    and, 38
Grounding, 116–118
    parent handout for, 211


H

Homework, contracts for, 121–
    123
HSQ, 57


I

IDEA; *see* Individuals with
    Disabilities in Education
    Act of 1974
Incentive programs, establish-
    ing, 74

Independence, increasing, 75–76

Individuals with Disabilities in Education Act of 1974, 68

Intervention; *see also* Family training program; Problem-solving communication training
justification for, 39–43

Interviewing
adolescent, 53–54
parental, 47–53
of teachers, 54–55

Issues Checklist for Parents and Teenagers, 58–62
form for, 196–198

**L**

Labeling, risk of, 51–52

Legal issues, 67–69
interview questions for, 169–170

**M**

Major Depressive Disorder, evaluation questions for, 185–186

Marital discord, instruments for evaluating, 64–65

Medical history, evaluation form for, 163–165

Medications for ADHD, 7

Mental disorder, defining, 41–42

Misbehavior
anticipating and planning for, 74–75
forms of, 18*f*, 18–19
minor, ignoring, 98–99
praising absence of, 101–102

Monitoring, lack of, 33

Mood disorders; *see* Anxiety/mood disorders

**N**

Noncompliance, defined, 17–19, 18*t*

Noncompliance/defiance continuum, 20–21; *see also* Defiance/noncompliance

**O**

Obsessive–Compulsive Disorder, 43

ODD; *see* Oppositional Defiant Disorder

One-on-one time, 97–98

Oppositional Defiant and Conduct Disorder, median age of onset, 30*t*

Oppositional Defiant Disorder, 1
criteria for, 21*t*, 50–51
differential diagnosis of, 44–45
discussing with parents, 83–86
evaluation questions, 173–174
family reaction to diagnosis of, 85–86
in parents, 63–64

**P**

Parent(s)
ADHD in, 63–64, 89
assessment interview, 47–53
depression and psychological distress in, 65–66
evaluation form, 169–193
and failure to reinforce positive behaviors, 32–34
inadequate management practices of, 36–37
management differences between, 52
marital discord between, 64–65
negative reinforcement by, 33–35
ODD in, 63–64
PSCT indicated for, 2–3
psychological characteristics of, 89

psychological disorders in, 42
questionnaires for, 46–47
temperamental/cognitive characteristics of, 38

Parent training; *see also* Family training program
screening families for, 69–70

Parenting, indiscriminant, 33

Parenting style, 90

Parent–teen conflict; *see also* Family conflict
defiant behavior and, 31–36

Peer relationships, measures of, 58

Penalties, use of, 110–111

Personality Inventory for Children, 56

Phobia, evaluation questions for
general, 178–179
social, 179–181

Physical abuse, reporting requirements, 68

Point system
completion of, 113–115
for contingency-management system, 106–107
parent handout for, 209–210
for penalties, 110–111

Positive attention, developing, 95–99

Problem solving
parent handouts for, 219–224
practice, 133–138

Problem-solving communication training
candidates for, 2–3
expected outcomes, 4–8
family reactions to, 132
family session in, 127–128
generalization of treatment gains, 9
goals of, 3–4

Problem-solving communication training (*continued*)
and individual meeting with adolescent, 127
introduction to, 125–132
Issues Checklist in, 128
maintenance in, 8
principles of, 75–79, 126
  adolescent involvement, 77
  communication skills, 77
  increasing independence, 75–76
  negotiable versus nonnegotiable issues, 76–77
  realistic expectations, 77–78
  respect for family structure, 78–79
professional background for, 1–2
program purposes, 1–2
rationale and steps of, 17–43, 129–132
success/failure predictors, 9–14
  child factors, 10–11
  parent factors, 11–13
  therapist factors, 13–14
Psychological distress, parental, 65–66
Psychological strengths, evaluation questions for, 191

Punishment
incentive programs preceding, 74
versus negative reinforcement, 34

**Q**

Questionnaires, 46–47

**R**

Reinforcement
negative, 34–35
  versus punishment, 34
positive, lack of, 32–34
Response cost, use of, 109–112

**S**

School advocacy, 119–124
  parent handout for, 212
School history, 49
  evaluation questions, 190–191
School Situations Questionnaire, 47, 57
Self-report behavior rating scales, 44
  adolescent, limitations of, 53
  for children, 57–58
  for parents, 62–66

Separation Anxiety Disorder, evaluation questions for, 181–182
Sexual abuse, reporting requirements, 68
Social Anxiety Disorders, 43
Social ecology, family, effects of defiance on, 28–30, 29f
Social phobia, evaluation questions for, 179–181
Social strengths, evaluation questions for, 191
SSQ; *see* School Situations Questionnaire
Stress, family, 89–90

**T**

Teachers
  interviewing, 54–55
  questionnaires for, 46–47
Teen(s); *see* Adolescent(s)
Teen noncompliance; *see* Noncompliance
Temperament
  parental, 38
  teen defiance and, 37
Tics, 49
Tourette syndrome, 49

**Y**

Youth Self-Report Form, 57